SPEAKING AT MEDICAL MEETINGS

a practical guide

James Calnan

FRCP, FRCS, DA, DTM and H, LDS, RCS, FCST

*Professor of Plastic and Reconstructive Surgery,
(University of London), Royal Postgraduate Medical School
and Hammersmith Hospital, London*

and

Andras Barabas

MD, FRCS

*Consultant Surgeon, West Suffolk Hospital,
Bury St. Edmunds, Suffolk, and Director of Clinical Studies at the
School of Clinical Medicine, University of Cambridge*

William Heinemann Medical Books Limited · London

William Heinemann Medical Books Ltd
23 Bedford Square
London WC1B 3HH

First Published 1972
Reprinted 1975
Second edition enlarged and revised 1981
Reprinted 1983

Illustrations mainly by Andras Barabas
Cover design by Cherry Calnan

ISBN 0–433–05001–2

*With no disrespect to the fair sex, the
male pronoun has been used
throughout. We realise that our writing
applies to both sexes, but to indicate
such continually is clumsy in English.*

Typeset by Method Limited, Essex
Printed and bound in Great Britain by
Redwood Burn Limited, Trowbridge, Wiltshire

CONTENTS

PART I: THE OCCASIONS

PART II: THE TECHNIQUES

FOREWORD TO FIRST EDITION

Medical meetings proliferate and form an increasingly valuable method of postgraduate education. Some go well in every way – they are organised properly but unobtrusively, the speakers are clear and concise, the visual aids are helpful, all the apparatus in the room works as it should, the discussion is forthright and constructive, and the audience leaves with a feeling of profit and elation. Others are painful to attend – the arrangements are chaotic, the speakers mutter and ramble interminably, the slides are illegible, overcrowded and irrelevant, the projection apparatus is out of order or mis-handled, the chairman takes no control of the discussion and everyone is left with a sense of frustration and of having wasted time.

A good meeting does not just 'happen'. The organisers, the chairman and the speakers must plan it from experience, according to principles which are now well established. Professor Calnan and Mr Barabas are highly accomplished performers and very experienced both in the art of speaking and illustrating their talks and in the craft of organising meetings. It is fortunate, therefore, that they have seen fit to share their expertise with us and that they have done so in such a practical, delightful and entertaining way.

This is a Do-It Yourself guide by professionals for amateurs. I am honoured to have been asked to write the foreword, for I have learned much and derived great pleasure from reading it myself. I have no doubt that many others will profit from it too. If its precepts are followed, all medical meetings will become enjoyable and educational occasions.

R. B. WELBOURN

Department of Surgery
Royal Postgraduate Medical School
Hammersmith Hospital
London   *20th September* 1972

INTRODUCTION TO FIRST EDITION

'Lectures were once useful, but now when all can read, and books are numerous, lectures are unnecessary'. **Samuel Johnson**

More than two centuries after Dr. Johnson's pronouncement, medical meetings still multiply and a visit to a lecture hall, as well as to a library, has become an integral part of life for most doctors. Books and journals abound, but in turn, an increasing number of conferences and symposia are advertised. The written word has not replaced the spoken; we all continue to read and listen. Also, our turn at the lectern seems to come more often. The slogan 'publish or perish' may soon be coupled with 'lecture or leave'.

Quantity does not imply quality: the present standard of speaking is deplorable. Much has been done to improve medical writing. Ill-prepared scripts are rejected by the journals, but can be read unchecked at conferences; editors exercise strict control over publications, but organisers of medical meetings give hardly any guide to speakers. Adjudicators and referees provide detailed criticism of submitted papers, but chairmen at symposia only murmur meaningless expressions of thanks after every talk, whatever its quality. Numerous books on good writing are available, but on speaking there are none.

Is the skill of speaking inborn or can it be acquired? This book is an expression of our belief in the latter. At the Royal Postgraduate Medical School, Hammersmith, where we both used to work, junior hospital staff take an active part in weekly conferences and discussions. Few appear born lecturers, but within months, through example, advice and criticism, improvement is obvious and gratifying to all. We shall try here to record in writing what we have learnt over the years by listening and lecturing. We hope this may be useful not only to junior doctors but to all who are called upon to talk in public. Yet our concern is not primarily for the speaker, but indirectly for members of the audience. We would like to bring the day nearer when they are not bored, confused and irritated by bad lecturing.

INTRODUCTION TO SECOND EDITION

In recent years, doctors have been given so much advice on how to improve their speaking that by now they must be either completely confused or completely enlightened. Another book on the subject can be justified only if it lessens the confusion without diminishing the enlightenment, which we hope the first edition of this small book managed to achieve. We now produce a second and enlarged edition with the same modest function: to serve as an inexpensive self-improvement guide for doctors whether teaching in the class-room or expounding at an international conference. It is mainly for the novice, but we hope that the more experienced lecturer will find something useful.

We have tried to keep to practical matters and have ourselves learned much since the first edition was published. We are grateful to those who wrote with constructive criticism and to those lecturers who have produced new ideas. Some sections have been expanded, with new material which seemed to us important: we hope they will be well-received. There has been new work on the physiology of public speaking, new ideas on do-it-yourself slides, on how to assess your performance and a clear need for detailed guidance to chairmen who can make or break a good lecture session. We realise that it may not be possible to turn everyone into a first class lecturer: some are 'reluctant lecturers' even though they have important things to say. But there is hardly anyone who cannot (with persistence, humility and a few guidelines) be prevented from being a bad or even poor lecturer. Kraft *et al* (1976) reported that at a meeting of the Association of Academic Surgery, in the USA, 66% of the papers presented were read (in our view this is cheating), that less than half of the slides were self-explanatory and, worse still, that the majority of speakers failed to transmit information effectively. What a dismal report! Yet we have the impression that the standard of speaking at meetings has improved in the past ten years; there is still a long way to go before all meetings show that high level of oratory and presentation worthy of medicine.

We both have one simply philosophy in life: enjoy what you do and if you don't then do something else. The philosophy applies to clinical practice, research, lecturing and to many other activities. We do appreciate that the first major lecture that anyone has to give may not be enjoyable until afterwards. We advise good planning, constant practice, a clear performance; the applause and congratulations which follow tend to tip the scales in favour for a repeat occasion. Lecturing can be fun, can be rewarding, can be worthwhile and, more importantly, all that preparation pays off; dress rehearsals before the day may be traumatic, but it is the day which counts.

Are lectures important in medical education? We think so. There is competition from electronic gadgets, but we do believe that the lecture has a major part to play. Any lecturer who can be replaced by a machine deserves to be. In much the same way that people fed on television flock to the live theatre, simply because it is different and real, so too will doctors welcome the chance to hear a good lecture. Lectures are given to make people think; it is our duty to teach our juniors to do so. One way is to stimulate others to ask questions, to argue a point, to contest authority – all in good humour, good logic and with the give-and-take of effective debate – but this can only be done if the lecture was clear, pointed and concise.

You cannot learn to play tennis just by reading a book. You can learn the rules, absorb the techniques, understand faults, but in the end you have to get out there on the tennis court and find out for yourself. At first, everything is strange however well-read you are and then things happen: improvement comes with practice. So too with speaking. Furthermore, habits of public speaking are changing; they should, as advanced teaching aids are developed and become available to all. The form of the traditional lecture cannot stay static, but must change with time. As the Red Queen (of Alice in Wonderland) said, we have 'to keep running just to stay in the same place'.

To the reader of this book we would say: pick it up and re-read a chapter or two, especially before you give your own lecture. If you don't agree with what we say, tell us. More importantly, make notes in the margin of your own copy; you are now on the way to producing your own book based on personal experience.

The prayer of the teacher of skills in speaking must surely be:

'Lord, grant me the serenity to accept things I cannot change,
The courage to change the things I can,
And the wisdom to know the difference.'

This is not entirely our view, but we do acknowledge our own limitations.

PART ONE
THE OCCASIONS

1

DEMONSTRATING A PATIENT

'The important thing is to make the lesson of each case tell on your education'.

Sir William Osler

At case demonstrations the junior doctor first encounters an audience. His conscientiousness in the preparations, his skill in presenting concisely a complicated case history and his tact in handling the patient can make his reputation. On the other hand, an indifferent disquisition, callousness towards the patient (Fig. 1) and an over-eagerness to impress, will become all too evident.

Case demonstrations vary from those at informal meetings of a dozen or so doctors, to those attended by hundreds in the lecture halls of postgraduate teaching institutions. From this wide spectrum we shall take two examples, one from near each end of the scale. In the 'Case Demonstration in a Minor Key', we imagine a busy general hospital, a small audience, and limited lecture hall facilities; for the 'Case Demonstration in a Major Key', we presume there will be a well-equipped lecture theatre and a large audience. To take the musical analogy further, first we shall have a chamber ensemble and then a full scale orchestra. The tune, however, will be much the same in both: it will be called by the presence of the patient.

Case Demonstration in a 'Minor Key'

Preparations

In selecting a suitable patient, the junior doctor should take the initiative. It is better to find and recommend a case of one's choice than to be asked, at short notice, to present an unfamiliar one. Successful demonstrations are usually on patients whose educational value has been recognised early in their management. The patient's permission must be obtained well before the event. Most patients enjoy and benefit from any extra attention, but Grann's (1965) warnings on 'The interesting patient syndrome', should be heeded: it is not permissible to over-investigate, to delay treatment, or to make the patient introspective.

Special attention should be paid to visual records, such as photographs or sketches of physical signs, of surgical operations, and of pathological specimens. The junior doctor should acquaint all concerned about his intention to present the patient. The radiologist and

3

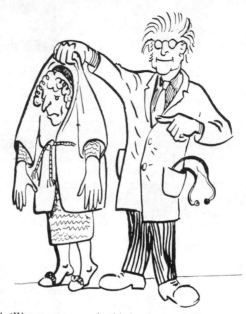

Fig. 1. 'Was ever woman in this humour wo'od' – *Richard III*.

the pathologist can provide enormous help, if warned in advance. The consultant in charge of the patient should also be informed and the general practitioner too, if he is likely to be in the audience. Finally, the relevant literature should be read and notes recorded on filing cards.

It is worth rehearsing (or at least estimating) the time taken for undressing and dressing the patient. You will have to decide what to do or say during this interval to keep the whole demonstration moving. Alternatively, a couch on wheels, with the patient prepared in an adjoining room, saves valuable time. Few lecture theatres have wall hooks for patient's clothes.

The Demonstration

The demonstrator must always remember that he is showing a patient, for information to the audience and discussion by the audience. It should not be a mini-lecture and therein lies the trap. The demonstrator will have read the relevant literature and, quite naturally, will wish to tell his audience all about recent advances (remember, some are not advances) in the subject. He is also likely to be THE authority

4

on the patient's condition at that time. Resist the temptation. If you, the demonstrator, have vital news to give, then slant the demonstration that way. For instance:

'In the textbooks, gallstones are said to occur in women who are fair, fat and forty: yet our patient is 21, dark and thin, so why?'. You can then lead the audience into questions and finally give your interpretation why it is important to understand that changes in diet, social environment, differences between countries, the changing scene, the adverse effects of textbooks on clinical diagnosis, new methods of discovery and so on, are important. Do not confuse your hearers at too early a stage between the differences on electrophoresis of lipoprotein II & IV. It's all a matter of judgement at the time. A mini-lecture destroys rapport with your audience, so don't do it! Demonstrating a patient by way of introduction to a lecture is an entirely different matter.

A case presentation should never be read (Fig. 2). Any medically qualified person should have the mental capacity to memorise a short case history, but a prompt card may be employed to remind one of the exact dates in the history and of the important results of investigations. The demonstration unfolds like a three-act play.

● The patient's name, age, her general diagnosis, the name of her

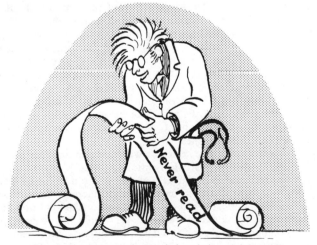

Fig. 2. 'An honest tale speeds best being plainly told' –
Richard III.

consultant and the name of the demonstrator, should be clearly written on the blackboard, for instance:

Patient 1, Mrs. Jean WHITE, 42, anaemia
presented by Dr. Smith for Mr. Sharpknife.

The demonstrator should not give the complete diagnosis (which was anaemia due to occult loss of blood from a carcinoma of the caecum), nor should he indicate in advance the outcome of the treatment; he should lead up to these, unravelling the case history like a detective story.

A brief introduction should explain why the case was selected for demonstration. For instance:

'The patient we are about to show you today is an unfortunate woman, who probably now has an incurable condition. When we first saw her a year ago the complete diagnosis was not made. We feel that we all have a lot to learn from this patient and we would like to invite your comments on her future management.'

● After the introduction the general plan may be as follows: the history of the illness is first told and the physical signs enumerated. At this stage the patient is brought in and introduced. Members of the audience now have the opportunity to question her for clarification of symptoms and examine her for the physical signs. After this the patient is thanked and dismissed. The provisional diagnosis is then established and the results of any special investigations disclosed.

In recounting the case history, irrelevant information should be omitted. Long lists of normal findings and the results of non-contributory investigations are boring, time-consuming and unnecessary. If any important omission is inadvertently made the audience will have the opportunity at the end to ask for it in the discussion. It is better to leave something out than to tell too much. Abbreviations should not be spoken; the term DVT may be used colloquially on ward-rounds, but in a demonstration it should be called, 'deep vein thrombosis'. In reporting the results of biochemical investigations, normal ranges should always be given. Few people in the audience will carry these figures in their heads.

● The demonstrator should conclude with a summary. This, like the introduction, should be short. For instance:

'We have presented today the case of a 42 year old woman who one year ago was treated for iron deficiency anaemia. Recently she developed abdominal pain and diarrhoea, and on examination had a fixed hard mass in the right iliac fossa. We would like to have your comments on her clinical course to date and your advice on her future management.'

A case demonstration should not last longer than 15 minutes and time must be allowed for the audience to question and to comment after the presentation. The demonstrator must not monopolise the discussion. He should be familiar with the relevant medical literature, but should not volunteer this unless he is asked to do so. Nothing is more boring and destructive to the success of a medical meeting than to have to listen to the demonstrator reciting, unasked, the relevant chapter of a textbook or of a recent article. To launch into a lecture after a case presentation is a grave and common mistake.

Visual Aids

All through this book we shall emphasise the importance of good visual aids. In a case presentation in the 'Minor Key' these may be difficult to marshal because time may be too short for adequate preparation and the venue of the meeting may be unsuitable or lacking in facilities. However, no such meeting should lack a blackboard, an X-ray viewing cabinet, and a couch on which to examine patients.

● The blackboard, with its easy availability and lack of need for preparation, is the visual aid 'par excellence'. As already stated, the blackboard should display the name, age, and general diagnosis of the patient from the start of the demonstration.

During the presentation, the demonstrator should use the blackboard to record the important dates of the case history and the results of salient investigations. He should also draw simple diagrams of the physical signs, of the temperature chart and of any surgical operations. These simple diagrams make demonstrations easier to follow and livelier, but to be successful, they must be planned and practiced beforehand.

● Nothing is more indicative of incompetent preparation than missing X-rays, or a desperate last minute search in the folder for the appropriate films. Having discussed the X-rays with the radiologist beforehand, the demonstrator should describe them himself. X-rays are often an integral part of the case history and to call in someone else to show them breaks the flow of presentation. The radiologist can always be asked to comment afterwards (we shall give different advice for case demonstrations in the 'Major Key').

An X-ray should only be visible to the audience when the appropriate stage is reached in the case history; this is best done by switching on the light behind the film already fixed to the viewing surface. The audience should not see the X-ray films beforehand, because these may distract their attention. For the same reason, films should not remain on view after they have been described. (Fig 3).

● The patient is the best visual aid, but also the one which requires the greatest skill in handling. Her safe and punctual transportation to the meeting, and her comfort while waiting outside the lecture hall, are the

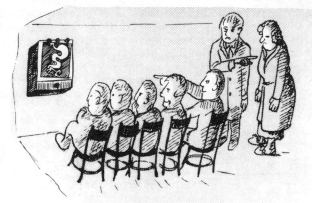

Fig. 3. 'Life is as tedious as a twice told tale vexing the dull ear of a drowsy man' – *King John.*

personal responsibility of the demonstrator. In front of an audience a genuine understanding of her as a person (and not only as an interesting case) and a sincere attempt to put her at ease, is appreciated. If she has been well prepared for the ordeal of facing the audience she will respond and give not only factual information, but reveal her true character; many mundane clinical meetings suddenly spring to life through the amusing or philosophical remarks of a patient.

The Advantages and Disadvantages of a 'Minor Key' Presentation

The main advantage is that the minimum of preparation is required and several patients can be seen within a short time. These may demonstrate different facets of one disease, or different diseases of the same system. Active participation by the audience is relatively easy; one or two individuals can be asked to examine the patient, to make a diagnosis or to give an opinion. If several patients are seen in one session, then it becomes possible for every member of the audience to take an active part. The disadvantage is that the use of audio visual aids is strictly limited and the lack of experts may reduce the value of the subsequent discussion which cannot thus rise to the level possible when demonstrating in a 'Major Key'. Because of this, the disease may not be placed in its true perspective.

Case Demonstration in a 'Major Key'

If, in a major demonstration, the patient and the demonstrator are considered as the soloists, the numerous experts in the large audience and the full gadgetry of a modern lecture theatre make up the orchestra. A conductor to create harmony is obviously needed. The conductor's – or chairman's – task, begins with the selection of suitable cases; he will also supervise the preparations for the presentation and he will control, firmly but unobtrusively, the demonstration and discussion.

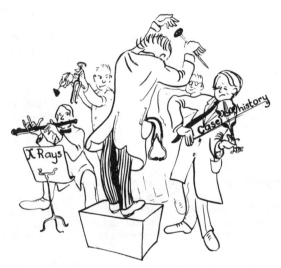

Fig. 4. 'Make heaven drowsy with the harmony' –
Love's Labour's Lost.

Selection of Suitable Cases

• Patients should be picked to match both the occasion and the interest of a particular audience. If the programme of the day includes a lecture, a patient may be chosen to complement it. Visiting guests contribute memorably to discussions, if the patients shown come within the sphere of their special interest.

• Patients presented may illustrate recent advances in diagnosis, or treatment; these may well make more impact than reading about new discoveries in journals. Full discussion can put these advances into true perspective.

- One learns more from mistakes than from successes. Complications of common methods of treatment should be highlighted; regrettably, failures are rarely shown and demonstrations are often used only to advertise successes.
- The showing of rare syndromes and the unusual presentation of a common disease benefit an audience, for many otherwise would never have had the opportunity to see them.
- It is permissible to aim occasionally purely at entertainment. An amusing case history, or a patient who reacts well to an audience, provides light relief in a succession of serious cases.

Visual Aids

For demonstrating in the 'Minor Key' we have recommended drawing on the blackboard; in the next chapter, on the short scientific lecture, we shall advise the use of lantern slides. Every occasion has its ideal form of visual aid and for the demonstration in a major key these are the epidiascope and the overhead projector.

The epidiascope is a versatile instrument; it can project typed script, diagrams, illustrations from books, pages of case notes, temperature charts and even trays of pathological specimens.

A large audience cannot discern details of radiological findings unless they are magnified. Projected lantern slides made of X-ray films could achieve this, but, for a case demonstration, the overhead projector provides a more appropriate method. By the use of suitable equipment the image of the X-ray film can be made to appear on the screen enlarged several times; shutters can exclude everything but the relevant part, so bringing important details into focus. A special indelible pencil can be used to point out and mark subtle pathological changes.

Other visual aids may be used. Close-up photographs of clinical signs, too small to be seen from a distance can be projected and may precede or follow the demonstration of the patient. A snapshot from a family album, predating the onset of the present disease (of, for instance, Cushing's syndrome or severe weight loss) and showing the patient in his normal environment provides added interest and a new dimension to the presentation. The blackboard remains a good standby, for illustrating surgical operations, or for impromptu sketches during the discussion.

The Discussion

The most entertaining and profitable part of a demonstration should be the discussion. Preparations for it must be made beforehand. Specialists in all the relevant disciplines should be asked to attend and must be briefed about the case; expert opinion on all aspects of the clinical problems should be available to the audience. Hence, for instance, the radiologist may point out all the detail seen in the X-ray and not merely that pertinent to the patient's disease. He can also explain the techniques used to obtain the views which he demonstrates and discuss the differential diagnosis from his investigations. Experts in other fields can explain the meaning and interpretation of special tests, and indicate the accuracy of these estimations – in biochemistry, haematology, bacteriology and immunology. They may look at the same clinical problem quite differently and this allows a cross-fertilisation of ideas. There is the opportunity to debate book knowledge as opposed to practical experience – in diagnosis, differential diagnosis, treatment, and subsequent prognosis.

Discussion can take place between experts so that areas of agreement and disagreement, or complete lack of knowledge, may become apparent to the audience. New ideas, new techniques in management and recent research, which may not yet have been published, can all be discussed. The clinical condition may also stimulate others in the audience to carry out research in this or related fields. The major demonstration may include distinguished visitors with other views and in this way dogmatism in one institution can be questioned. It also demonstrates to a wider audience that many doctors in different fields are concerned in the management of one patient – and clearly to her advantage; such a demonstration of unity of purpose keeps everyone up-to-date and on his toes. Indeed, the debate may be of great calibre. Unfortunately, complete rehearsal beforehand is virtually impossible; hence the quality depends largely on the excellence of the individual speakers.

The Chairman's role in calling on the various speakers has already been likened to that of a conductor, but unlike a piece of orchestral music a discussion should never follow a rigid score. The Chairman should not divert contributors into a preconceived pattern; impromptu speeches and spontaneous remarks, the 'thrust and parry of argument', are the life blood of good discussion.

Perhaps the best recipe for successful discussion is to insure that the standard of presentation is consistently excellent. This will attract a large regular audience, with a variety of expertise and talent, which in turn will generate, unaided, a good discussion. The Chairman's main duty will thereby be reduced to simply calling on those who wish to speak and eventually bringing the proceedings, reluctantly but firmly, to an end.

The Ten Special Values of a Demonstration

1. You can show a rare disease, in the flesh. Your audience having seen and heard will never forget the condition – and thirty years later may startle all around by the accuracy of the diagnosis for another patient. The Ehler-Danlos Syndrome and the Treacher-Collins Syndrome come to mind: once seen, never forgotten.

2. It is a live performance. In the same way that most of us yearn for the theatre as a relief from films and television (where a sense of unreality exists) so too do doctors. After all we do see, talk to, and treat individual patients: slides and lectures never quite replace the personal confrontation.

3. The patient may disclose unexpected information of importance, often because she has never been asked a particular question.

4. The patient can show her own innate sense of humour and so contribute something which the demonstrator cannot. Many patients do. Who could fault the remark of one patient who said 'Reports of my death are greatly exaggerated'?

5. The audience can question the patient and confirm for themselves the statements made by the demonstrator.

6. Patients can be asked how they feel about the treatment they are receiving, and so disclose unreported side-effects.

7. The history of world events, recorded by a patient who took part, is enlivened by his personal observations and so adds a new dimension to an otherwise mundane occasion.

8. The demonstration allows the audience to fit all those biochemical investigations and X-rays to the person concerned.

9. The audience can examine patients, make their own diagnosis and be questioned.

10. When demonstrating, the demonstrator discloses his relationship with the patient, his clinical ability, his humanity and his professionalism; all of which can be instructive to the audience.

Duties of the Demonstrator

To conclude this chapter we would like to point out that the demonstrator has certain duties to his patient, for which he alone is responsible.

1. He should obtain the patient's permission for the demonstration and explain exactly what is required.

2. He should not over-investigate the patient, delay her treatment, nor delay her discharge from hospital to facilitate the demonstration.

3. He should organise her safe and punctual transportation to the place of the meeting.

4. He should introduce the audience to the patient by saying who they are and the patient to the audience by correctly pronouncing her name and where she comes from. This is no more than good manners, but it does engender respect towards the patient and the staff.

5. He must cause no physical pain to the patient by allowing others to feel a tender area.

6. He must cause no mental anguish to the patient by the use of words which carry serious connotations.

7. He must defend the patient's self-respect at all times. A good relationship between the patient and the treatment team must surely be the foundation on which educational demonstrations are built.

8. He should make a point of thanking the patient publicly at the end of the demonstration and reinforce the gratitude of the audience privately afterwards.

9. Finally, the demonstrator has a duty to the consultant in charge of the patient who should always be allowed the last word – as a courtesy and for simple justice. Often the management of a patient will be criticized – implicitly or explicitly – and the consultant must be allowed to explain. In a court of law, counsel for the accused is allowed to speak last before the judge sums up (in our case the Chairman) so why not at a demonstration?

2

THE SHORT SCIENTIFIC COMMUNICATION

'The scientific man is the only person who has anything new to say and who does not know how to say it'.

Sir James M. Barrie

What the case demonstration is to the houseman, the short scientific communication is to the registrar: it is his main opportunity for public speaking. Yet the two occasions are utterly different. Case demonstrations often have to be prepared in a hurry, but there is usually plenty of time for the preparation of a scientific paper. At a case demonstration the atmosphere may be casual, the audience composed of friends and acquaintances, but at a scientific meeting the proceedings are formal, the audience largely unknown and critical.

For the young registrar preparing for his first scientific communication a lot may seem to be at stake. The subject may concern the results of careful investigations made over several months, or even years, the impact of which can be ruined by bad presentation. Also, perhaps for the first time, he will be 'playing away from home', representing his research team or hospital. His chances of promotion to a higher post, if not actually dependent on his performance, may at least seem so to him. How is one to help him in his unfamiliar role as a lecturer?

Firstly, he should realise that he will not be communicating some earth-shattering discovery. But the audience will be interested in incomplete work; they will be only too keen to help the lecturer answer his unformed question: 'Where do I go from here?'. Secondly, the lecturer should aim to interest his audience, not to impress them: they will soon spot the difference.

Thirdly, fine prose should be ditched in favour of clarity and direct speech. Euphony of the words spoken is a bonus of liquid gold: it solidifies when appreciated. The Welsh have a knack of using musical speech; so did Bernard Shaw's dustman – I'm waiting to tell you, I'm wanting to tell you, I'm willing to tell you (the order may be wrong, from memory, but matters little: the statements are somewhat repetitive, but the song is there).

Fourthly, the short scientific communication imposes a strict discipline on the individual. We all appreciate the good lay-out of a written report: it looks more attractive, is easier to read, quicker to understand, and carries conviction. The same applies to a lecture, but is not so obvious. Lecturing is an art (and a craft that can be learnt) and therefore a very personal matter. No two people will talk alike on the same subject: each will have a different point of view, a different way of expressing the same facts, a different vocabulary. We all speak differently because we are different. But, for the short scientific communication there is an imposed code of conduct. The lecturer has to:

1. describe the facts,
2. put the facts in the correct logical sequence,
3. state the facts in plain English, so that all may understand,
4. provide supporting facts with adequate information and illustrations,
5. make a reasonable conclusion from, an interpretation of, his work which is warranted by the information provided. The conclusions should be itemised so that everyone in the audience knows what the speaker has discovered, inferred, or recommended.

Fifthly, as soon as he has been invited to give a lecture he should jot down on the back of an old envelope the title and any ideas he may think of at the moment. These notes will later be transferred to several sheets of paper and the whole organised under the three structural headings of introduction, main theme, and concluding remarks. It is often valuable to compose a title sentence, and in this way concentrate thought on what you wish to say.

At this stage the lecturer should be clear what he has been asked to do:

1. to review a subject,
2. to report on research,
3. to provide practical instruction, or,
4. is there complete freedom to range within his speciality?

The lecture plan will be slanted differently for each.

There is no point in hoping for inspiration, for a miracle on the day, when you can so easily put all your energy into making it come right. Talk to friends, take advice, but do end up in the library where essential information is stored. Speaking well in public means thinking well in private. Isaac Newton when asked how he solved difficult problems, answered 'by thinking about them continuously'; such advice applies here. While preparing for a short scientific communication the lecturer has to do a great deal of thinking, planning, preparation and practice.

It helps to appreciate that there are three separate stages in its production:

1. The collection and selection of data.
2. The arrangement: getting the structure right and deciding on the most suitable visual aids.
3. Polishing, writing it out and rehearsal.

The Collection and Selection of Data

Gathering the material for a short scientific communication is usually a problem of selection and of compression (Fig. 5). By the time a lecturer is invited to talk at a scientific meeting he has more than enough to declare and his main task is how to say it within the given time limit – usually 10 to 15 minutes. Obviously, he will not be able to disclose all that he knows and he will have to select that part of his subject he regards as best worked out and the most original. He will have to look at his own research work critically and decide which portion will make a coherent 10-minute story.

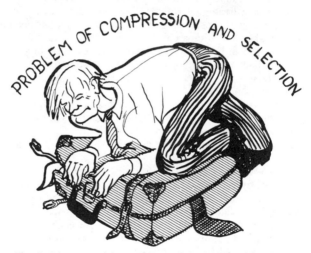

Fig. 5. 'I know a trick worth two of that' – *Henry IV, Part I.*

For instance, in a study of the rate of gastric emptying, he may decide to leave out his findings on patients with gastric pathology and concentrate instead on the normal, comparing his methods and results with those of previous workers. Thus, by narrowing down the field to methodology and normal physiology, he may make his short talk more complete and more interesting than if he tried to cram all the available facts into it. The temptation of the novice is to overload; it should be resisted. He should also remember that what is left out is not lost; it may form the topic of a second lecture for the future.

The Arrangement of Data

This consists of two parallel parts: getting the structure right and choosing the appropriate visual aids. The two go hand in hand. In a short scientific communication, visual aids are essential. Complex matters have to be put over within a limited time and this would be impossible without tables, charts and diagrams. The only practical aid is to project slides; there are usually good facilities at scientific meetings and there is enough time to prepare them beforehand. In this book a whole chapter is devoted to the preparation, design, use and storage of slides. Hence, only a broad outline is given here and the accompanying diagrams summarise the overall plan of the structure of the lecture and of the arrangement of slides.

The Structure

The structure of the lecture is dependent on three parts – the introduction, the main message, and the conclusions.

• The introduction should be delivered with the lights on and hence the street lamps in Fig. 6. The lecturer is introducing not only his subject, but, figuratively, himself. The audience will want to see him and will want to get used to his shape, voice and mannerisms. Even at a scientific meeting a few seconds have to be allowed for such apparent trivia. The first few sentences are the most important and often the most difficult to get right; commonly they are the last to be found and composed in writing the script of a lecture. They should never be read and no visual aid should accompany them. What is wanted is a 'punchline' which will immediately alert the interest of the audience.

After a few sentences, rarely more than 2 or 3, the first slide will be asked for and the lights will be dimmed. They should not come on again until after the last slide. Asking for 'lights' half-way through loses precious minutes and irritates the audience.

When asking for 'the next slide please' change the pitch of your voice so that the request is separated from your lecturing voice. Alternatively, you can nod to the projectionist, and so demonstrate good team work (but do remember to thank him afterwards).

The first slide should relate to the introduction; yet, it must be simple and appeal to the common denominator of knowledge in the audience. For instance, in a lecture on gastric emptying, which may report work using radio-isotopes and a computer, one could start with a diagram of the stomach or an X-ray of a barium meal.

• The main message of the lecture demands that the ideas are in sequence. The facts must be so arranged that the next idea flows naturally from the first.

It is unwise to introduce a new idea more often than once every 2 to 3

17

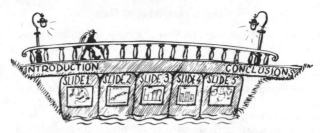

Fig. 6. 'Too swift arrives as tardy as too slow' – *Romeo and Juliet.*

minutes; hence, in 10 minutes probably no more than 4 new ideas can be presented. The purpose of a short scientific communication is to propose an hypothesis, to describe the observations which were made to test it and to present a conclusion. This is the nub of the matter.

All this means that the usual detail concerning material and methods, as in a written paper, has to be abandoned. An outline, the bare minimum for comprehension, is all that can be accomplished. Besides, the audience is mainly interested in the results of the work and no great detail is required. The lecturer should inform and try not to bore the listeners with irrelevant matters.

Each and every one of the main ideas should be illustrated by a slide. Thus, as the theme of the communication unfolds, a steady flow of slides will accompany it and in a 10-minute talk, there will be time for no more than about 6 to 8 slides in all. The integration of the spoken and visual components must be perfect. This implies that a slide will have to be projected exactly when it is referred to and stay on the screen only for as long as its content is being explained. To achieve such co-ordination a great deal of polish and rehearsal will be required.

• The conclusions should stem naturally from what has already been said. It is a good idea to summarise briefly what you have already told your listeners and then to enumerate the conclusions you have drawn from the work as you make them. If you have been using lantern slides and the last one has your conclusions on it, try not to finish in the dark. Ask for 'lights' and have a few final phrases to say when you are clearly seen and can re-establish rapport and identify yourself with the audience.

The Illustrations (With an Example)

Every lecture can be summarised in a list of headings and once this is done a suitable illustration should be found for each. The task, therefore, is two-fold: first a search for the basic ideas and then an attempt to turn these ideas into visual images.

This process is best explained by the use of an example. Let us take a paper from the journal 'Surgery', (1971, Vol 71, p. 157) on 'Bile as a gastric secretory stimulant', by Nahrwood and Hershey. The main facts in this paper were as follows:

● What others have said: reflux of bile from the duodenum to the stomach occurs in man.

● The questions which the present work tried to answer:
   (a) Does bile stimulate gastric secretion?
   (b) What is the mechanism by which bile acts as a stimulant?

● The design of the experiments:
   (a) Four dogs with both innervated and denervated gastric pouches were used.
   (b) The innervated (antral) pouch was perfused with acetylcholine, concentrated gall-bladder bile and hepatic bile.
   (c) The acid output from the denervated (fundic) pouch was collected every 15 minutes and measured.

● Results: In each dog 3 experiments and 16 readings were made, a total of 192 measurements.

● Conclusions:
   (a) bile stimulates gastric acid secretion;
   (b) this stimulation must be mediated by a hormone, probably gastrin.

Let us now find the illustrations. For the first, the fact that there is reflux from the duodenum, something simple and eye-catching is required. A radiological technique has been developed to show this reflux during duodenal intubation; hence, a slide could be made of an X-ray film showing it.

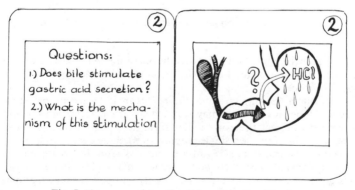

Fig. 7. 'Assume a virtue if you have it not' – *Hamlet.*

19

Next, the two questions posed should be illustrated. A verbal slide projecting them word for word onto the screen is not the right solution. A better plan is to depict the first two of them diagrammatically (Fig. 7.) The diagrams will have minimal labelling and so will only make complete sense if accompanied by a verbal explanation. An important principle thus emerges: the speaker should not put on the screen precisely what he will say, but use his slides like diagramatic maps, so simplified that they need the spoken word to explain them (Ollerenshaw, 1962).

Now we turn to the third heading, the design of the experiment. The lecturer may be tempted to use photographs of the operation for construction of a gastric pouch. It is more than likely that these will fail to explain the procedure; simple line drawings will be clearer and more effective. Such diagrams are too complex for a single illustration, and so should be made into two separate slides (Fig. 8).

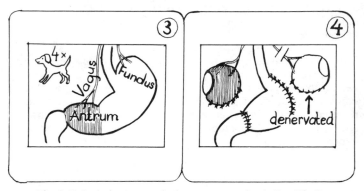

Fig. 8. 'I do desire we may be better strangers' – *As You Like It*.

To make the important point that the operations were carried out on animals, the silhouette of a dog is, therefore, added to the first of the two diagrams.

The fourth heading contains the results in 192 separate measurements. Unbelievable as it may seem, there are lecturers who would attempt to project these in tabular form, like pages from a railway time-table, or even use a single graph with so many curves on it that it resembles the tracks in snow of a popular ski-run. It is better not to show tables at all, nor to crowd the results on a single graph, but to go straight to one group of experiments only and plot them as a graph. (Fig. 9)

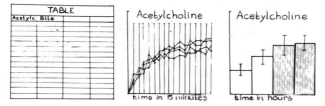

Fig. 9. 'The daintiest last to make the end most sweet' –
Richard III.

Of the five agents used to stimulate gastric acid, acetylcholine served as a control because it is known to produce a gastric acid response. Two things became clear from the central graph in Fig. 9. First, that there was a similar response in all 4 dogs and so there is no need to show all 4 curves, and secondly, that there is a gradual increase in the acid response reaching a plateau in the third and fourth hours. We could now construct similar graphs for the other stimulants, gall bladder and hepatic bile. These curves would be similar to the ones for acetylcholine in that the results agree in all 4 experimental animals and a plateau of maximal response is reached, in every case, in the third and fourth hours. There is, therefore, no need to show these graphs at all as they do not answer the question posed in this paper, namely, 'Does bile stimulate gastric acid secretion?', and 'What is the mechanism?'. A histogram or column chart to compare the responses to the three stimulants serves a better purpose (see slide 6 in Fig. 10).

We have, therefore, planned 7 slides in all:

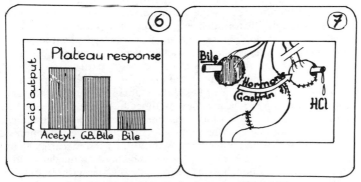

Fig. 10. 'Truth has a quiet breast' – *Richard II.*

21

1. An X-ray to show reflux to the stomach (which is not illustrated here).
2. Diagrams to ask two questions (Fig. 7).
3 & 4. Diagrams to illustrate methods (Fig. 8).
5. A histogram to show the typical plateau response by gastric acid.
6. A histogram to compare the gastric acid responses to acetylcholine, to hepatic and to gall bladder bile.
7. A concluding diagram (Fig. 10).

Repeated rehearsals with the preliminary sketches of these proposed slides will soon show whether they are suitable or otherwise and such rehearsals will also integrate the verbal and visual components of the lecture.

To conclude, let us list some of the general principles demonstrated by this example (and for further examples, see Zollinger and Howe, 1964).

● First, prepare a list of the main facts to be presented in a lecture.

● Then design the slides to show each of these facts.

● Try not to display on the screen exactly what you say; make the visual and the verbal parts complementary, not overlapping, never conflicting.

● If you have a table as an illustration, try a graph instead; if you have a graph, substitute a diagram – in other words, strive for simple and apt pictorial illustrations.

● Finally, never overload, and from one good slide always try to make two (or more) better ones.

Polishing, Writing it Out, and Rehearsal

All short lectures and speeches should be written out in full because time is not on the lecturer's side, and because detailed writing is an invaluable discipline. This is creative writing in which any talent for artistry can be disclosed. If the lecture is written out then it can be revised thoroughly before delivery; the grammar can be corrected, verbal errors erased, phrases made more pointed and the visual complement dove-tailed to the spoken word. If an authoritative statement is being made, this must be word perfect so that no alternative interpretation may be put on it; for this, the only practical way is to write it out in clear detail. One great advantage is that the written lecture can be rehearsed several times and rehearsal can start at an early stage of preparation; it is thus easier to practice timing, gestures and intonation. The exercise of writing alone will impress words and phrases on the memory, without the need to learn it all by heart. Finally, it is easier to make notes to be used on the day from a complete script. Although we advise writing out the script in full, we emphasise that a short communication should never be read.

Early Practice

For this the sketched diagrams are spread out on the floor and the provisional script read aloud. A tape recorder and a clock should be at hand even at this stage (Fig. 11). Practice reading aloud: it will be strange at first, but you will soon learn how to use your voice. Read the lesson at church if need be.

A great deal of redrawing and rearrangement of the diagrams, rejection of unsuitable material and experimentation with new ideas, is often required. This is the really creative part of planning a lecture; hence, an alert mind and undisturbed surroundings are essential. Family, friends, television and indeed all distractions, should be banished from the room and from the mind.

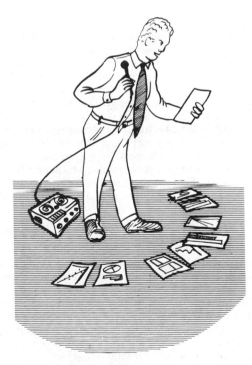

Fig. 11. 'Though this be madness, yet there is method in't' – *Hamlet*.

Intermediate Practice

The script begins to take shape and the number and the sequence of diagrams have been decided. This stage should be reached more than three weeks before the day of the meeting and now is the time to rehearse with friends, with the family and with colleagues. Their criticism should be sought and accepted. Only after exposure to several pairs of critical eyes should the sketched diagrams be passed on to the medical artist or to the photographer; the lecturer can be curiously blind to glaring errors and omissions in the design of his own slides.

Remember that the art of giving a good lecture depends largely on humility in inviting good and early criticism and help. Nothing is more annoying for the artist and for the photographer than having to reproduce slides in a great hurry because the lecturer's original designs were discovered to be inaccurate only at the final rehearsal.

Final Practice

Many institutions require their members to deliver important public lectures to their own colleagues before the actual meeting. On such occasions the lecturer should be word perfect and have a complete set of slides so that they will, in essence, be 'dress rehearsals'. We are all editors (or should be) of our own lectures. Every time we change a word we are editing the script. Some are reluctant editors and it shows in the final product. Editing your own proposed lecture is an essential step in improving its quality; but it is only the first step. Independent judgement by a third party, or better still (and more daunting) a rehearsal before all your colleagues helps even more.

The object of a dress rehearsal in public, which must be held at least two weeks before the final day to allow time for alterations, is to check:
● The timing of the lecture under real conditions, with slides, and using a stop watch,
● Any technique of delivery which requires amending,
● What questions are likely to be asked, and,
● The confidence of the speaker.
A last minute rehearsal in public is usually valueless to the speaker: he has not enough time to incorporate constructive criticisms.

The rehearsal audience should:
● Spell out criticisms. Nobody wants constructive criticism (it's all we can do to put up with constructive praise) but it must be endured;
● Justify their remarks, and the lecturer should stand up to justify his own presentation;
● Stress the major errors of presentation;
● Be impartial in criticisms;
● Be constructive by offering alternative techniques.

In this way we learn to do better ourselves while training others to be better than us. It is not easy.

A. E. Shephard has proposed a Speaker Index for assessing the quality of a lecture, which we have modified and reproduce later. His proposals have merit in that it is possible to score other people's lectures and so reflect on your own performance.

On the question of the 'meat' of the lecture, here is a more detailed check list for the lecturer (and for the rehearsal audience):

1. Is the aim of the lecture clear?
2. Is the problem defined? The purpose stated?
3. Are all questions answered?
4. Are all the necessary elements to interest and to inform the audience during the introduction included?
5. Is the material presented in the best order?
6. Should material be added or removed?
7. Are any statements contradictory?
8. Is it worded effectively and accurately?
9. Are there enough or too many slides?
10. Is the title too general/too wordy/inaccurate?
11. Are there too many or too few references to previous work?
12. Is the pace adjusted to the complexity of the material?
13. Is there sufficient explanation of complex ideas?
14. If several authors are involved have they been given recognition?
15. Is the lecture a complete unit without obvious jumps in changes of direction?
16. Is there redundancy?
17. Will the theme be remembered?
18. Could you do better?

Thereafter, it is important to continue to rehearse privately for 5 to 10 minutes at a time, right up to the day of public delivery. You will gain confidence and find that gestures and emphasis come naturally; you will also by then have a better inflection in your voice and will know the introduction and conclusion by heart. All the minor defects in the earlier presentation will be smoothed away. As Bacon noted: 'No remedies cause so much pain as those which are efficacious'. We would add that the joy of efficiency, seen and heard, erases all previous pain of preparation. When the day comes this lecturer will be confident, knowledgeable and well-rehearsed.

The Day of the Lecture

On the day of the lecture, a final look at the numbered slides to check that they are in correct order is advisable before surrendering them to the projectionist. The lecture hall and its facilities should also be observed ('Case the joint' is always good advice), so that there will be no last minute fiddling on the podium with the microphone, with the pointer, or with the signalling apparatus.

The lecturer should walk in front of his audience like a professional boxer into the ring, ready for an ordeal, but knowing that he has done all he could to get himself into the fittest and best condition, through weeks of careful preparation. He should carry no script for he is not going to read; all he may carry in his hand are one or two small prompt cards. (Fig. 12).

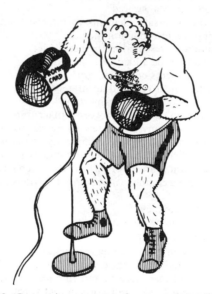

Fig. 12. 'Come, give us a taste of your quality' – *Hamlet*.

The easiest advice in the world to give is also the most unhelpful: 'Don't worry about it!' Experienced speakers will know that it is just this apprehension which constantly keys them up to give a good performance.

Before leaving the subject we would like to comment on two features which the lecturer will think about after his lecture. The first is nervousness and how can it be overcome; the second is on methods of self-assessment of performance.

Nervousness

Anyone who has had to speak in public for the first time will remember how he felt – rapid pulse, thumping heart, dry mouth, sweaty brow, trembling hands, a desire to micturate, the fear of failure, a certain hoarseness of voice. In other words, all the symptoms of anxiety, which can begin well before the time of the lecture. The intensity of, and the nature of, the individual speaker's reaction depend on his personality, experience, general health, the subject of his talk, and the audience: In modern jargon, the 'emotional barrier'.

The extent of these changes in normal physiology, in otherwise fit young people, has been reported by Taggart, Carruthers and Somerville (Lancet 1973. Volume 2. pages 341-346); 17 doctors speaking at medical meetings and 13 laymen (seven with coronary heart disease) when speaking at various occasions, were studied immediately afterwards.

The findings were surprising:

● All had tachycardia, with the fastest heart rate reaching 180 beats per minute: the mean maximum rate was 151 which settled to 120 during question time.

● The electrocardiogram showed abnormalities in the QRS complex. Only one of the healthy subjects had depression of the S-T segment (a sign of ischaemia), but three of the seven with known coronary disease developed this abnormality; and in a further three patients, who already had S-T depression, this deepened while speaking.

● Ectopic beats, sometimes prolific and often multi-focal occurred in a quarter of the healthy subjects and were common in those with coronary artery disease.

● Total catecholamine concentrations increased in most speakers, almost entirely due to a raised noradrenalin concentration (the adrenalin levels were unchanged, possibly because as the speaker proceeds his mood changes from acute anxiety to a less insecure feeling).

● Plasma free fatty acid concentrations increased by 30%.

● Plasma triglycerides increased 25% (due to endogenous synthesis), but the cholesterol levels were unchanged.

● Increased systolic blood pressure, in keeping with the increased heart rate.

Taggart, Carruthers and Somerville then gave fifteen subjects a single oral dose of 40mg oxyprenolol one hour before they were due to speak – and managed to prevent the cardiac and biochemical changes recorded above. They therefore suggest that beta-blockade by a single dose of an appropriate drug will alleviate these unpleasant symptoms, but warn that freedom from side-effects of the intended dose should be tested beforehand on a less important occasion.

Our advice is simple. We do not advise beta-adrenergic blockade, except perhaps for those with known coronary artery disease. We would advocate good preparation, plenty of practice and suggest that the symptoms of anxiety may be beneficial even for the experienced speaker. Many people speaking in public do not have unpleasant symptoms beforehand; we suspect that this may well be due to experience and training. In the same way that an athlete must train for every competition – and he knows when he is not fit because he too suffers – so must the lecturer if he is to give of his best; like the athelete, he will be drained of energy after the event but will soon recover. The non-physical stress of a lecture is equivalent to moderately vigorous exercise; joggers please note.

Methods of Assessment

All along we have tried to convey one simple message for a successful lecture: obtain the interest of the audience and hold it: buttonhole every person by your opening remarks and never let go. The experienced speaker recognises this achievement by three things.

Firstly, there is absolute silence. If you have never experienced this before it can be unnerving. It is immediately recognisable by all five senses: it is the taste of power, the smell of success, the feel of mastery, the sight of victory, and the sound of conquest. No one in the audience moves, coughs, or speaks to his neighbour; you have the undivided attention of the audience.

Secondly, all eyes are on you and all ears tuned to hear the next word. Everyone is listening to you and you know it. Unfortunately no one can remain still for long, so either you allow the audience to relax or wait for them to do so: the former is better because you retain control. A longer-than-usual pause in speaking, asking for the next slide, an indication of change of direction in the lecture (for instance: 'now let's consider the real evidence') or a simple directive to the audience such as 'You can relax now because I'm not going to persue that subject further' – all these help.

Thirdly, applause is the only appreciated interruption. When we attend or watch competitions, such as ice-skating or ballroom dancing, we expect the judges to provide a numerical assessment for finding the winner. The same 'close marking system' is used in the English FRCS final examination. So why not a numerical method for judging objectively the value of a lecture? If we can apply the method to others, then why not to ourselves?

There are three methods for self-assessment:

The Speaker Index

David Shephard, a physician at the Montreal General Hospital, Canada, published his 'Speaker Index' as a guide for the assessment of the skill of communication from judging papers given at medical meetings (Brit. Med. J.: December 1979 p 1403-4). Shephard's argument is that doctors are not taught how to communicate, don't know how to assess their own performance or that of others, and so they use subjective rather than objective values. We have modified his rating chart and produce it here. It is a score card of five judgements: bad (1), poor (2), good (3), very good (4) and excellent (5). The obvious thing to do is to use it at the lectures you attend. In this way score 3 or the 'average' becomes identified with your own personal assessment. From there you can begin to appreciate how good you should be. The listener makes his assessment and mean score from eight primary characteristics in part one, the minimum that should be completed. Part two serves two purposes: to identify the many items that go to make up each primary characteristic and to permit of an optional but comprehensive rating. The SPEAKER INDEX (or mean score of performance) may thus be derived from calculating the total score in

Part 1: Rating of primary characteristics of the lecture

Name: _____

Title: _____

Date: _____

	Score					
Characteristic (low)	1	2	3	4	5	(high)
1. Speaking ability						
2. Personality of the speaker						Total score =
3. Use of language						(Max. 40 points)
4. Relationship with the audience						
5. Content of the lecture						Mean score or
6. Management of the environment						Index =
7. Audio-visual aids						(Max. 5.0)
8. Suitability of title						

Part 2: Details

(low) (high)
1 2 3 4 5

1. SPEAKING ABILITY
    A. Articulation/ pronunciation
    B. Volume/pitch/ tone
    C. Rate/rhythm
    D. Emphasis/gesture/ animation
    E. Spontaneity/ ad-libbing

2. PERSONALITY OF THE SPEAKER
    A. Dress
    B. Confident/ relaxed
    C. Interested/ sincere/friendly
    D. Enthusiastic/ inspiring
    E. Humour/wit

3. USE OF LANGUAGE
    A. Direct/plain/ familiar words
    B. Informal/ personal
    C. Precise/concise
    D. Correct
    E. Variety

4. RELATIONSHIP WITH THE AUDIENCE
    A. Naturalness/warmth/ courtesy
    B. Eye contact
    C. Audience interest
    D. Audience rapport
    E. Management of questions

(low) (high)
1 2 3 4 5

5. CONTENT OF THE LECTURE
    A. Facts/Depth
    B. Organisation/ structure
    C. Documentation
    D. Importance/ interest
    E. Time-keeping

6. MANAGEMENT OF THE ENVIRONMENT
    A. Command of space (stance, posture, mannerism)
    B. Control of acoustics
    C. Control of lighting
    D. Control of projector
    E. Control of screen

7. AUDIO-VISUAL AIDS
    A. Visuals — quality
    B. Visuals — quantity
    C. Visuals — usefulness
    D. Audio
    E. Exhibits

8. SUITABILITY OF TITLE
    A. Accuracy
    B. Meaning
    C. Effective
    D. Clear
    E. Concise

part one, preferably with close attention to part two. Simply make a cross in the score column opposite each item. Join these marks with a line to gain an indication of the general pattern (that is a 'profile') and finally, add up the total scores and divide by eight to give the Index.

We are inveterate lecture-goers (others prefer opera). We try to keep our ears open for good phrases to use and our eyes for illustrations with impact. We steal all unashamedly and have made assessments of 92 lectures during the past five months. The results are less disturbing than expected. With a total possible score of 5.0 points, the average mean score was 3.1. Hence, 20 lecturers were bad, 30 were average, 30 good, and 12 excellent. This is very much a personal view. The trouble is that when we talk about objective measurements (of say pronunciation, rate and rhythm) there are no exact standards by which to compare. Spontaneity and ad-libbing are qualities dependent on experience, a quick mind, and the nature of the speaker. So, to a large extent, good lecturing depends on subjective assessment, as does any live performance on stage or in the market place. The best performers were natural actors with a good script and appropriate props (usually slides, for slides are the common currency in lectures although like currency they may be counterfeit).

The 'Speaker Index' chart may also be used, with suitable modifications, to assess the performance of chairmen at symposia. We believe that this kind of measurement is a step in the right direction and should be fostered. Indeed, a group of doctors analysed the performances of speakers, chairmen and audiences at the Fifth Annual Convention of the Medical Societies of Greece (Tsakraklides *et al.*, B.M.J. 1980 iv. 1194-1196), to find that 'most chairmen failed to comply with simple rules of procedure and with the expectations of speakers and audience'. Although the method of scoring differs from that published by Shephard, the conclusions agree that the interest of the audience was affected by the performance of speakers and chairmen. These findings, we suspect, apply world-wide. Moreover the fact that 62% of the Greek speakers depended almost entirely on their manuscript for a ten-minute talk, compared well with Kraft's 66% for a meeting in the USA, even though the methods of assessment differed. The problem of effective communication can be recognised, whatever the means used to disclose it.

Audio-Videotape Recording.

With modern television developments it is now possible to buy a videotape cassette recording machine at a reasonable price. There has to be extra lighting on the speaker, who must wear a radio microphone, but the whole lecture can be recorded and re-run – preferably in private with the speaker and his instructor only, certainly for the first viewing – so that points of technique (good and bad) can be demonstrated. This teaching aid is still rather experimental; for longer than a ten-minute lecture it demands a lot from the teacher. But it may prove its worth in due course; we don't know, but from experience of other 'modern aids', we suspect that it will be a tedious and time consuming method.

The biggest single advantage is that you actually see yourself on the

31

screen: and that is the only way to find out how you appear to others. The effect may be horrifying. For the first time, speakers see their personal tics (blinking, nervous smiles, mannerisms, shifty eyes, lack of sincerity – and a great deal more to destroy the self-image). Speakers can judge for themselves whether they come over as sincere, truthful, trustworthy types; or as pompous, flippant, shady neurotic zombies. And that monotonous voice!

The Video-cassette recorder (VCR) allows all this to be revealed. You need not believe what you see, but it is advisable to believe and try to improve. The speaker must wear a lapel microphone and be well lighted so that he may not even be able to see the audience, sometimes a blessing, but it will make him sweat a bit. There are many systems and a choice of black-and-white or colour, but colour must now be the system of choice. Before buying it is advisable to see both, do some hard thinking, and decide what can be afforded; to pay dividends the VCR must be used constantly and some form of assessment devised (see the Speaker Index).

Tape Recordings Only.

It is fairly simple to set up your own tape recorder during a lecture and to record what you say and how you say it. But you cannot stray too far from the microphone. Alternatively the recorder can be worn under the suit on a suitable holster, and the microphone placed on a lapel of the jacket. By this means it is also possible to pick up questions from the audience during question time, and their reactions, but the great nuisance is extraneous noise. Even so, to learn that you have said 'um' 20 times and 'er' 16 times during a ten-minute dissertation is worthwhile information – and not all that easy to correct.

3

THE GUEST LECTURE

'To lecture well, that is, with profit to your listener and without boring them, requires not talent alone but experience and skill'
Anton Chekov in *A Dull Story*

We give advice on the art of lecturing with some diffidence. The rules of a case demonstration and those of a short scientific communication are fairly well defined, but a recipe for a successful 50 minute lecture is less easy to discover. Indeed, it may differ from speaker to speaker. In the longer lecture the content and the personality of the lecturer will always be much more important than the skill of the presentation. We can remember, for instance, listening enthralled to the reading of a script (something we in general deplore), by someone obviously unused to public speaking and unaided by a single illustration – yet, the impact was enormous. The originality of the message and the sincerity of the speaker mattered more than the sophistication of delivery. However, we know neither how to develop a fascinating character nor how to acquire something unique to say. Our aim, therefore, is modest: to advise the average doctor on how to become a better lecturer.

Some General Principles.

Know What you have Have Been Asked To Do.

The lecturer must be clear about what he has been asked to do, because the lecture plan will be quite different for each:

1. to review a subject,
2. to report on his research,
3. to provide practical instruction,
4. to describe recent advances,
5. or, is there complete freedom to range widely in the subject of his choice?

Generally, the invited lecturer will be given some indication of what is required. If not he should correspond with his host until all is clear and not accept until then. We have been embarrassed on several occasions by lecturers who spoke on subjects which had little to do with the advertised title. Of all human attributes, communication is the most frail. If there is doubt after much letter-writing, then telephone to get this important aspect sorted out. We emphasize again, that no lecturer should accept an invitation until he is clear in his own mind what is required and what the host expects.

THE LECTURE INVITATION

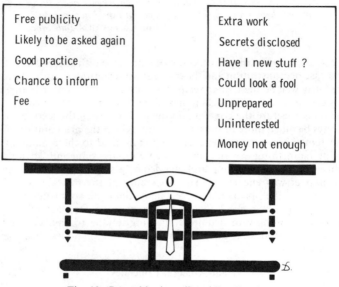

Fig. 13. 'By and by is easily said' – *Hamlet*.

The Four Aims

The four aims of a lecture should be to:

    entertain,
    stimulate,
    inform,
    teach and persuade the audience to act.

The proportions of the mixture will depend on the audience, the subject, the occasion and the duration of the lecture. If time is limited, it may be possible to provide only a frugal portion of each, but we believe that all four aims should be included.

Think About the Audience.

In his fascinating book *Most Secret War* Professor R.V. Jones had this to say:

'Subconsciously I acquired the two secrets of lecturing from which everything else follows: first, to believe that you have something worth telling your audience, and then to imagine yourself as one of the audience . . . You must, for example, talk in terms that appeal to the background experience of your audience. You must be audible at the back of the room, where the details of your lantern slides must be visible and your blackboard writing legible; and you should not distract your audience with antics and fidgeting. You must also detect by the change in tension when you are in danger of losing its interest'.

We echo his advice that the lecturer should try to imagine himself as one of the audience in the back row of a crowded lecture hall.

For a lecture, one always has some idea who the audience will be and so you must try to answer six questions, before planning a single word, and think about your audience:
1. What will amuse them?
2. What will be of particular interest?
3. How much can they absorb?
4. What do they need to know?
5. What do they want to know?
6. What makes them tick?

How Much Can You Put Across?

In planning the lecture, the greatest constraint is time. So, what can be put across clearly within the allotted time? Usually remarkably little. Planning therefore concentrates on making the best use of time. The successful lecturer will ask himself two questions:

1. *What can a lecture do better than the written paper?*

(a) Anything one can look at can make a statement in seconds rather than the minutes required to describe it. Hence the lecturer with advantage, can show patients and a series of clinical photographs.

(b) Opinions based on experience come over well in speech.

(c) The lecturer can argue for and against a certain hypothesis or a line of management, in a way that no journal editor would tolerate.

(d) Real understanding can be imparted in elementary terms which might be considered too juvenile for a journal. For instance, in describing the I^{125} fibrinogen test for the detection of deep vein thrombosis, the lecturer can describe how isotopes are made and detected, how two different isotopes of the same chemical may be identified separately. In this manner, some of the audience may really understand the subject, perhaps for the first time.

(e) Research which may be unfinished or have negative results (and will, therefore, never be published) and research already completed, but not due to be published for a year or more.

35

(f) A bit of philosophy: new ideas and new hypotheses always provide the personal flavour to a well thought-out lecture.

2. *What can a publication do better than a lecture?*

Again, there are at least five things and all are to be avoided, so discard the lot at the planning stage and not during the lecture:

(a) Tedious details of methods.

(b) Complicated tables and graphs.

(c) Fine prose which is lost when spoken and better replaced by enthusiasm and animation.

(d) Closely argued description particularly of apparatus which is difficult to put over anyway, and,

(e) Most statistics which are rarely understood and when not understood leave a sense of doubt which is the last thing you want in a lecture. In the written paper, authors can be consulted and the value of their work assessed by correspondence. In a lecture there is rarely this opportunity even at question time.

The Lecture Title

The host will demand a title for the lecture early on so that he can advertise it widely. It is worth writing a title immediately you have been asked to speak, as a kind of true North for your subsequent planning, later to revise it as thoughts crystallize and then to reply to your host. Heresy in the title often goes down better than conformity. Be controversial in the lecture, but try to indicate this in the title.

Some use titles to amuse, to puzzle, to challenge and even to attract an audience. But the title must be informative to the audience you wish to speak to. The effectiveness of a title can be assessed by answering five questions:

1. Is the title correct: does it accurately represent the subject?

2. Does the title state or imply the limits of the subject?

3. Does the title mean what it says and is it understandable?

4. Has the title been expressed as succinctly and as effectively as possible?

5. Does the title have punch?

Many lecture titles do not stand up to these criteria, because they:

1. Contain deadwood. Length is no guarantee of precision or clarity in a title. The non-informative phrases such as 'a study of . . . an investigation into . . . a report of . . . the analysis of . . .' usually contribute nothing. Leave them out.

2. Are vague. Vagueness obscures meaning, so change 'A method for measuring creatinine in urine' to 'Measurement of urinary creatinine by electrophoresis'; 'A system for improving community care' to 'Preventive medicine in a South London Community'; 'The

effect of stopping smoking on coronary infarction' to 'Stopping smoking reduces heart attacks'.

3. Use single words. For instance the title: 'Lasers'. Does this mean all types of lasers in all forms of surgical procedures? Or was the lecture intended for physicists only?

4. Are long and cumbersome. Even if the title contains no worthless phrases it may still be too long for easy understanding, so chop it into two parts: the first the main theme, the second the limitation. For instance, 'How bile is produced and some experiments in man and animals' would look better as 'Bile production: human and animal experiments'. 'Day-care Surgery: organisation and purpose' is better than 'The organisation and purpose of day-care surgery' because the first title has greater impact and is more direct than the second.

Planning

A lecture is planned and delivered as a single offering. Its structure is simple. The attention of the audience must be captured by the first sentence uttered and then held until the end. Too many people worry about what to say, but forget that they have been invited to speak because they are recognised experts in the subject and should have something important to say. The composition of the main message of a lecture, then, is usually a matter of selection and compression. Because you have something to say you were invited, so why not settle for four aspects of your subject:

THE LECTURE PACKAGE

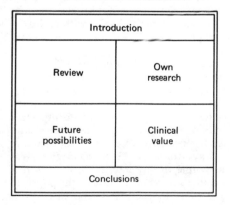

Fig. 14. 'We must take the current when it comes, or lose our venues' – *Julius Ceasar*.

37

What's new in research?
What are the clinical applications?
What are the difficulties and unwanted effects?
How's the future?
Hence you must:
emphasise the subject,
present it in the most effective form,
put it together neatly (you will know too much anyway and have to do some radical surgery to make your contribution palatable). Use linking sentences to join up each aspect of the subject. The final result will be a smooth flowing lecture script.

To describe how a lecturer should set about collecting his material would mean to outline a whole way of life, including the steady and ceaseless accumulation of observations not only from research, but from clinical work and from reading of the related literature. Without the continuous input of fresh and personally acquired information, there can be no worthwhile output in the form of instructive and lively lecturing.

We all know the fossilised lecture, delivered by someone who stopped making any intellectual effort a long time ago, and year after year resurrects the same old topic – the result of some youthful research. The script has a musty smell, the slides are faded and dusty; he arouses no enthusiasm because he has none himself. We cannot condone this type of lecturer and the only hope for him and for his audience is that he will not be asked to talk again. On the other hand, enthusiasm and inquisitiveness are not enough. When the time comes to prepare for a talk, the lecturer may find that he cannot remember exactly where he has read the relevant articles and may discover that his interesting cases also came and went, without leaving so much as a clinical photograph or a slide made of their unique findings as a souvenir.

A filing system and a collection of personal slides are required; in short, the discipline of regularly recording and of storing information. Consultants with secretaries and willing registrars may delegate much of this work, but the habit must be acquired at an earlier age, while still struggling on one's own as a junior. On storing slides we shall give advice later; on filing references, the actual method is not as important as the perseverance with it. The best method, therefore, is the easiest and that is always to carry 13 × 20cm filing cards and write immediately a resumé of any interesting articles read. These summaries may be quite short but the title of the paper, the name of the journal and the exact location, must be carefully noted for easy retrieval in the future. A good adjunct or alternative, is to keep torn-out articles (of one's own journals!), request reprints or have photocopies made. If one is to invest in a filing cabinet – a good idea – a large one with hanging lateral files is practical. A more expensive, but in many ways more convenient system, is the circular, revolving rotafile.

The times of regular observations and recording will be interspersed with bursts of greater activity. These should not coincide with the need for preparing an instant lecture. They should arise when the accumulated facts suddenly seem to suggest a new idea. In addition to regular browsing of the journals the prospective lecturer will now start to read in depth. He may even formulate an hypothesis and put it to test in an experiment or in a clinical trial.

When the time for giving a talk arrives, this lecturer will be bursting with enthusiasm and fresh facts to relate to his audience, and there is no better prescription for success.

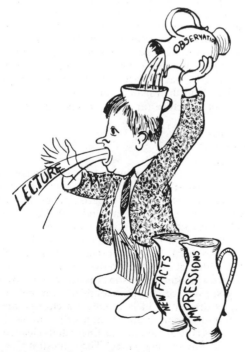

Fig. 15. 'Wherefore are these things hid' – *Twelfth Night*.

Structure of the Lecture.

For anything longer than a single case report, a formal presentation in writing is expected: often called the IMRAD structure – that is Introduction, Material and Methods, Results and Discussion. Nothing less is acceptable and there are advantages for the writer and reader. Each section can be composed piecemeal, perhaps with a long time-interval between; each can be altered, rewritten and have its own illustrations and references. The reader is able to scan any one section and, if satisfied or stimulated, may then read all; he does not have to and will not wade through pages of detail which do not interest him.

General Outline.

A formal lecture too, has a structure. It is much simpler than that of a written paper and does not intrude on the text. Nor are the subdivisions so obvious. The major constraint is temporal – the beginning and ending are at predetermined times (or should be) and the total duration is limited. The audience is largely known, if not by actual name at least by designation; hence some interest and knowledge of the proposed subject can be presumed although both may vary widely. The speaker will have been chosen to attend and not be self-invited. The competent lecturer will make enquiries of his host to satisfy himself that he has an accurate mental picture of what is expected from him, and then plan accordingly.

The structure of a lecture (as we have said before) is relatively simple:
1. Introduction;
2. Main message;
3. Conclusions.

Indeed it is so simple that many lecturers fail to understand what each section involves. Worse still, they do not realise that a lecture is a live performance, such as acting in the theatre, giving an after-dinner speech, or even unveiling a memorial, and that lack of rehearsal is immediately obvious to the embarrassed audience.

The *introduction* introduces the lecturer and his subject. He has to make himself known simply because most of the audience will not have seen him before, although they may know him by reputation. All will be interested to see what kind of person he is – tidy or untidy, what age, a good-looking speaker or an ugly mumbler, immobile or a caged animal, a snappy dresser or in last century's clothes, any peculiar mannerisms, truthful and accurate, humble or pompous, credible or fringe? Do his shoes squeak and are his finger nails clean, is he clean-shaven or bearded, bald or long-haired? These questions may not even be asked or answered consciously, but there is ample indication that until the cerebral cortex of each member of the audience is satiated with such trivia, the owner may hear but he will not listen.

Next, the subject has to be introduced in such a way that the attention of the audience is immediately captured. The introduction therefore has to be in simple terms, in easily understandable language, so that everyone is alerted and wishes to hear more.

The second item, that is the *main message*, causes much trouble. The lecturer has been invited because he is an expert in his subject – and therefore knows too much to tell within the time available. He must leave a lot out and the only way to do this is by ruthless trimming. It is generally accepted that one new idea every 2 minutes is as much as even the most intelligent audience can absorb. Moreover, absorption is not the same as understanding. It is wise to severely limit the various aspects of your subject in the lecture, perhaps to concentrate on special features of diagnosis, to highlight the results of some recent personal research, to explain how both of these have influenced clinical management, and to end with speculations about the future.

The *conclusions* should follow naturally and quite obviously from what has been said earlier. They should not require statistics to make them evident or even credible.

Logical Order.

The audience will not understand information flung at them randomly: a bit of geography here, a piece of research there, a funny story tossed in for good measure. Instead, they require that the subject be reduced to some understandable scheme. Careful organisation of the material is the key to a successful lecture. To the listener, clear and straightforward order reflects clear and straightforward thinking. A muddled lecture suggests a muddled investigation, whether true or not. Hence, organisation of a lecture is important because it relates directly to timing. Perhaps it is better to define a lecture as the briefing, the evidence, and the evaluation. The lecture should flow easily from one phase to the next, and the whole must provide a complete package; this applies as much to a ten-minute lecture as to an hour-long dissertation.

In medical terms we could describe the structure of a lecture as:
1. The Skeleton:
   the main message you wish to put over. Like the human skeleton it should be upright, and easily recognisable
2. The Muscles:
   clothe the bare bones and give power to the argument
3. The Skin:
   covers the whole, makes the shape and size visible to the

least interested member of the audience and gives the entire lecture a distinctive form.

The lecture should always have a formal structure: beginning, middle, and end. We have laboured the point because this is the first rule. How you organise it, that's your prerogative. For instance, in reporting on research you can give the results before you discuss how you went about discovery. The central idea is to tell a story which will interest your audience. In analytical lectures, the beginning is the premise or hypothesis, the middle is the analysis, and the ending is the synthesis. In describing a new device, the beginning is the review of the methods and mechanics of others, the middle is the presentation of the details of your device, the ending is the summing up of its advantages and disadvantages. Hence there are three sections:

Briefing
Introduction.
Supply preliminary information the listener requires to understand your message.
State the problem, define or explain existing facts.

Evidence
Objective report of new facts that bear directly on the subject.

Evaluation
The summing up of the evidence (as in the Law Courts).
Give recommendations, a summary, or conclusions.
Indicate where more work is required.

Order and simplification are the first steps towards mastery of a subject and the chance to gain the complete attention of your audience. Use the blackboard, if you must, to focus attention on what you intend to talk about; or use a slide, but you will lose your audience in darkness thereby. We would suggest that no lecturer is a speaking machine programmed to a specific topic; he should be free to use his imagination to produce a new, fresh, invigorating lecture which will be remembered by the majority.

Specimen Headings for a Lecture.

1. *Introduction*

   Statement of problem.
   Statement of purpose.

2. *Analysis of Published Work*

   Assumptions.
   Calculations.

3. *Experiments.*
    Procedure.
    Equipment.
    Special tests.
    Results.

4. *Discussion of Results.*

    Comparison with published work.
    Comparison of theoretical and experimental results.
    Opinion about general application of results.
    Conclusions.

But do make sure that:

1. the manner in which the parts are organised will be apparent immediately to the audience;

2. you proceed always from the familiar to the unfamiliar; Establish a common ground with your audience; if you don't they will soon be lost and you will be disappointed;

3. you determine whether description or diagram (usually a slide) will serve your purpose best;

4. you check your pace according to the knowledge of the audience. If in doubt, slow down.

Other Ways.

There are many other ways of arranging an interesting lecture, while still getting away from the formal structure of writing. Rudyard Kipling wrote a short verse, as introduction to his book *The Elephant Child*:

> I keep six honest serving men
> They taught me all I knew.
> Their names are what and why and when,
> And where and how and who!

Based on this poem, the lecturer can debate evidence and opinion as six questions: what should be done? Why should it be done? When should it be done?, and so on, In reviewing medical and surgical procedure these headings can be quite effective; they need not be taken in the order provided by the poem.

We believe it important that the lecturer should use his imagination and creative instinct to experiment with various types of structure; some will be winners, others flops; some will be appropriate to a particular subject, others not. No matter. Variety is the spice of life and variety is the spice of form. We advise that the lecturer should never, if possible, give an identical lecture the second time: minor or major changes will provide freshness for the lecturer and his audience.

The Introduction.

The introduction consists of two parts: the opening sentences and the introduction proper. We shall deal with them in reverse order.

The Introduction Proper.

Many speakers have trouble with the introduction to a lecture because they don't know:
1. exactly what the introduction should do for the listener,
2. how to determine what the audience already knows,
3. how to organise their material effectively.

What should the introduction do?

The introduction to a talk, lecture or demonstration should do four things:

1. Supply preliminary information to help the audience understand and appreciate the real message quickly, by outlining what the talk is about, for how long, and that there will be time for discussion afterwards.

2. Stimulate the interest of the audience by challenge, question, quotation.

3. Prepare the audience intellectually and emotionally for the serious job of listening to what you have to say.

4. Establish a relationship between audience and speaker.

What does the audience already know?

The answer to this question derives from what you know, or think you know, about the audience. When asked to lecture on any subject you should find out beforehand as much about the likely audience as possible. Hence, if lecturing to members of the Department of Surgery at a hospital, will there be consultants, registrars, house officers, medical students and nurses present? What proportion will know anything about your particular subject? How keen will the interest be? If lecturing to general practitioners the audience may be fairly homogeneous in their knowledge, but not necessarily in their interest in your subject. If talking to a club, will children and adults be present?

Specialty	D	What people in your specialty know
Subspecialty	C	What surgeons know
Professional	B	What doctors know
General	A	What everyone knows

For some audiences you will have to define technical terms, for others such would be resented.

The diagram of a pyramid serves as a guide to planning the assessment of audience knowledge.

So pitch your introduction at the appropriate level.

How should you organise the material of the introduction?

We can turn the pyramid upside down to lead the listener from the familiar to the unfamiliar, from the general to the specific, and so allow him to interpret and evaluate your particular topic.

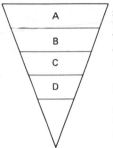

A	Statement of general knowledge: what is known and what is unknown
B	What you intend to talk about and what you will omit
C	Possible hypotheses
D	How you set about discovery
	Subject to be expanded in the lecture
	Main body of the lecture

● **The Opening Remarks**

The first few words should grip the audience and arouse their curiosity and attention. This may be achieved by a variety of ways:

1. By a bold, challenging statement which may be highly controversial, but later, in the course of the lecture, is qualified, explained or altered until it becomes acceptable ('I do not believe that vagotomy has ever cured a patient with peptic ulcer').

2. By asking a rhetorical question, or questions, to which the talk will gradually attempt to give the answers ('Is duodenal ulcer a psychosomatic disease?' 'Should we try to help the whole person rather than his ulcer?').

3. By making use of some topical event to draw a comparison between it and the seemingly unrelated subject of the lecture.

4. By recounting a relevant personal experience, ('Last month I was in . . .').

5. By using a quotation from antiquity, or the long forgotten past, to put into historical perspective what is to be presented as a recent advance.

6. By stating an informative but little known fact which is of special importance to the audience.

7. By the ridiculous remark. For instance:

'I have done many foolish things in my life, but perhaps the most foolish has been to come and talk about a subject to experts in the field of . . .'

On one occasion a nervous young man at the Surgical Research Society, seeing the first two rows of professors, licked his lips and started: 'Ladies and Gentlemen, there are many people who know more about this subject than I – but, as I don't see any of them present, I will begin'. He gave easily the best paper and went on to qualify as a doctor. Our laboratory technician did well by realising the importance of never being afraid to be himself and that he probably was the expert in a subject he had been steeped in for some years.

8. By a simple statement of fact about your subject ('Pain, jaundice and loss of weight are the most frequent symptoms of cancer of the pancreas. Jaundice can be relieved by quite a minor procedure, but pain . . .')

In some instances, the statement may highlight the subject in a way that the audience may not have thought about before. For instance: 'In order to survive in a hostile environment, we need to have intact immune defenses which can destroy infecting micro-organisms and parasites. Given a few days to mount an immune reaction, most of us can repel an infection even of a virulent kind'. The lecture was on immunology, but the introductory words made the subject of personal interest to every member of the audience.

9. By making a reference to previous speakers (by name) and their contributions. Such an opening requires an alert mind at the meeting and cannot be rehearsed beforehand. But it does help to pull together different aspects of the subject under discussion and shows that you have been listening. If previous speakers have been heard before, you probably know roughly what they will say and so can make an outline of your own remarks: you can state that you agree or totally disagree with what has been said – be controversial, but never offensive. To tie your presentation to what has been said already (in a symposium, for instance) it is essential to attend the whole session; you may have to omit part of your own script to avoid duplication and be briefer than intended, a bonus for the audience.

10. By a mysterious or intriguing statement: 'Yesterday hardly anyone had ever heard of it, today everyone is talking about it. I mean of course the subject of . . . '. Then develop ideas from this and either expand the subject or focus down to one particular aspect to be treated in full later. 'I am probably one of the very few gynaecologists who works in a chastity belt' (his consulting rooms were in the same street

46

as two convents, as he explained later).

11. By tape-recorded music. Why not thirty seconds from the ballet *Les Sylphides* to introduce a lecture on chronic leg ulcers? Or something from Sibelius' Fifth Symphony – and then begin to speak: 'that rumbustuous music was written by the 19-year-old son of a well-known doctor in Finland. Today no one remembers the doctor, everyone the son. Memorable and dramatic music but, not nearly as dramatic as the patient who falls down dead from pulmonary embolism in the middle of a crowded ward'.

The tape recorder can provide voices and noises by way of introduction. All the lecturer has to do is to say 'listen!' and then switch on. It might be thought a gimmick, and should not be used too often unless the lecturer wishes to earn the reputation of being the local disc-jockey.

12. The homely, 'Let me tell you a story. A story of intrigue, bad judgement, bad thinking, bad practice, but with a happy ending. It is the story of the management of . . . '. People listen to stories, so tell them a story relevant to the audience and the subject.

The possible variations for the opening remarks are numerous, if not endless, but they must be strongly worded to carry maximal impact. A lecturer should not run timidly into a lecture theatre, like a rabbit, or hide behind false modesty. If he is really convinced that he has nothing worthwhile to say, he should have declined the invitation to speak.

The Main Body of the Lecture

● Audio-Visual Aids (Illustrations)

We compared the short scientific paper to a bridge supported from end-to-end by a succession of pillars, in practice, a set of lantern slides (Fig. 6).

This would not be our advice for a 50-minute lecture. Occasionally, an exceptionally interesting collection of pictures may hold the attention, but more commonly a monotonous succession of slides in the darkened lecture theatre induces sleep after half-an-hour. Slides, therefore, should not play an exclusive role in illustrating a lecture. The 50-minute talk should resemble a river, rather than a bridge: it should flow from one scenic effect to another. Every sweep of this flowing stream should open up a new vista; there should be a surprise around every corner. In other words, a longer lecture requires change and variety to hold the interest of the audience and this can be partly provided by a good assortment of visual aids. We suggest four.

The Blackboard.

After referring to it in the makeshift setting of a minor case demonstration we return to the blackboard in the much more formal surroundings of a lecture. We recommended it for the case demonstration because of its availability and lack of need for preparation. Now we would like to point out a different potential – its dramatic value. Using a chalk, the lecturer is free to gesture and move about, yet he remains the focus of attention. He may add, wipe off and alter his drawing while proceeding with his explanation: the sketch becomes a dynamic and integral part of his talk. Also, as the lecture unfolds, the keywords and main headings should be written on the board. Thus, at the end, a short summary of what has been said will be displayed, giving a visual skeleton of the whole lecture.

Wallcharts, pathological specimens and patients.

These may also be used. A chart has much more impact if it is only revealed when referred to and not displayed beforehand. The drama is to unfold it before the audience. Also, a pathological specimen should be produced only at the appropriate moment, almost the way a magician pulls out a white rabbit from his top hat. Patients may be introduced, as surprise guests are in a television show. The lecturer should borrow some of the techniques, if not the gimmicks, of professional entertainers.

Not all adjuncts need be visual: the recorded voice of a patient with myxoedema remains, to one of us, an unforgettable part of a talk on disease of the thyroid gland.

The Tape Recorder.

In another chapter, we discussed the value of a small portable tape recorder in practising for a lecture. We advised a relatively cheap piece of equipment which could fit into a jacket pocket and would be constantly available: the quality of the recording mattered little. Here, we wish to advise on the value of a more expensive tape recorder, one which is still easily portable (and therefore battery operated, with an option to use the main electrical supply to save your pocket and produce greater volume) and will have an output of at least one Watt.

Too few lecturers make use of modern facilities, such as the tape recorder, to introduce or conclude a lecture, to illustrate in sound a feature which will come over well by this medium. The instrument has several uses: for it can demonstrate better than by any other means:

1. Music, to show qualities of the composer pertinent to the lecture: even as 'mood music' it has a place (where words fail, music speaks – Hans Christian Anderson).

48

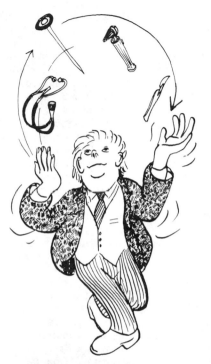

Fig. 16. 'It is meat and drink to me to see a clown' –
As You Like It.

2. Children's voices, for a lecture on paediatrics, perhaps to pick out one voice and then demonstrate that particular patient.

3. The sound of towns, the noise of motor cars and trains, to illustrate the background of living in a city.

4. And, by contrast, to demonstrate the sound of the countryside, birds, animals.

5. Accents and dialects, of different geographical areas.

6. The speeches of famous people, to illustrate almost at first hand their views on current problems.

7. The differences in languages and how modern medicine, increasingly international, has to find methods of communication in order to treat disease under difficult circumstances.

8. Certain diseases, such as those affecting the central nervous system (and others, for instance myxoedema as already mentioned)

can be diagnosed quickly and simply by hearing the patient talk. There are also a number of other speech defects which record well on tape and these will add a new dimension to a lecture.

Recording on tape is not just for the enthusiastic amateur. The machine can be taken to a clinic in the hope of recording something of value. You may be lucky, but most recordings require strict editing if the final product is to have impact. When the patient reads aloud a set piece, the interviewer can then read the same script on tape to demonstrate any differences. The script should be short (less than one minute). Such a method is most economical of time and labour because the audience will recognise the voice of the lecturer without difficulty and so appreciate quickly what features they are supposed to spot. There are several other uses for tape recording and we recommend you to list your own particular opportunities. One is to use it for planning a journey by car: instead of having to stop and read a map, you can switch on for further instructions (having recorded them the night before) and therefore make your route easier to follow. You can record notes for meetings to attend, items to deal with, ideas to follow, jobs requiring action, all within the comfort of a motor car while travelling to work. You can also, of course, rehearse your lecture (to the consternation of other drivers) and play back until you get it right. A tape recorder is a wise investment, but do use it constantly.

The tape recorder should not be used as a 'gimmick', but as an essential part in the story you unfold. It is the 'audio' part of audio-visual aids. Admittedly, the speaker is the most important audio-visual aid for any lecture, but even so people have failed to recognise the value of recorded tapes. On the other hand, quotations from books or articles should be read from the original: the opening of a book and the change of intonation while reading aloud will add spice to a spoken lecture.

Slides and filmstrips

If slides are used they should not be scattered in ones and twos all through the talk, with consequent switching on and off of the lights. They should be shown in one or two uninterrupted sequences. One possible solution is to leave them to the end. Well designed and attractive pictures will entertain just when the concentration of the audience is beginning to flag. Short film strips can be used the same way, almost as a reward for sitting through and listening to a lecture. The audience can be told early on that illustrations will follow later. The expectation and anticipation of these create, one hopes, better concentration, even during the earlier, unillustrated and more demanding section.

Lantern slides may be used in three different ways:

1. as a peg to hang the lecture on, often as word slides or fairly simple and pretty pictures: on the whole we do not advocate this;

2. to support the spoken word, concept or idea, by re-inforcement in a visual way;

3. to show something which the audience, perhaps, have never seen before.

We can summarise the different visual aids needed:

Blackboard
Overhead Projector } to support the spoken word.
Lantern slides

Films
TV } to provide a visual experience of movement.

Audio-tape } to aid visual imagination.

● **The Story**

We have, in this chapter, described the overriding importance of the content of a lecture, advised on the choice of visual aids, and emphasised that the speaker should begin and conclude strongly. One might think that little more need be said about a lecture and that from these good sources it will flow successfully and carry the audience with it, like a river carries a pleasure boat. Unfortunately, this is not the case. Care must be taken in the selection and arrangement of the ideas. In a written paper there is a standard formula: introduction with reference to previous works, details of materials and of methods, results and discussion.

In a lecture the same plan will rarely work. The nature of a live presentation demands a less divided and less jerky narrative. Technical details and masses of data may be absorbed when reading, but in a lecture they are out of place and confusing. The main ideas only need be presented and, if necessary, references can be given for further reading. The function of the lecture is to entertain, to survey wider fields, to arouse interest and even enthusiasm. The acquisition of detailed factual knowledge must be left to quiet solitary study. The steady sequence of ideas should carry the theme of the lecture like giant pylons carrying a high voltage cable.

Educational research also shows (Beard, 1968) that maximal attention is obtained from an audience in the first 20 minutes of a longer lecture. The complex and attention demanding parts should be concentrated, therefore, into the first half; the second half should be more leisurely, used for illustrations and explanations with examples. Indeed, from this point of view, a lecture can be compared to a mountain walk which starts with an uphill climb and finishes with a downhill stroll. This simile completes the allegorical landscape of our lecture: the flowing river with interesting and varied sites on its bank, the well-distanced march of electric pylons over the horizons and the up-and-down slopes of a single mountain.

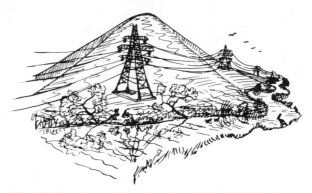

Fig. 17. 'Smooth runs the water where the brook is deep' –
Henry VI, Part II.

Closing the Lecture

Keep your lecture flowing, gently, alter the pace, alter the interest, alter the stress; change from fact to fiction, from emotion to candour, but do keep going. In effect, this means no interruptions, no long pauses, and so no asking for 'lights' halfway through the lecture which will only break the continuity of the lecturer's speech and destroy the concentration of the audience.

Yet, while part of the lecture can be taken at a leisurely pace, the concluding remarks should not. Don't dawdle to fill out time, but neither rush to get finished as though you had had enough of the subject. The conclusions from a lecture should be spoken clearly and crisply at a moderate pace so that the audience can take them in, and prepare their own questions.

Do not:
1. end weakly,
2. add any new information,

3. make it an anti-climax by adding unimportant detail or irrelevancies,

4. go on too long,

5. use cliches such as 'one last word', 'I would like to add', 'I repeat again'.

A lecturer must introduce and conclude, not just start and stop talking. The beginning and the end, although relatively short, take a disproportionate amount of time in preparation. They have to be composed carefully and memorised word for word, while the rest of the lecture need not be fully scripted and may be, to a certain extent, improvised.

Anyone can stop speaking, but only a lecturer can finish. Lecturing is an art no matter how prosaic its subject, and nothing is so fatal to a work of art as a failure to complete its form. This completion is often achieved by a return to the first statement. If the introduction contained a controversial pronouncement it can now be qualified or even retracted; if the speaker began by asking questions he now may attempt to give his final answers. This circular form is a pleasing device and it so clearly indicates to the audience that the end has been reached.

There are other ways to conclude:

1. By using signal words such as 'finally' or 'in conclusion'. Say 'finally' once only; to use the word more than once is not just an abuse of language, it also disappoints every member of the audience who, expecting you to wind up, will be annoyed to hear you rambling on five minutes later. If it has been a dull lecture, raising the hopes of the audience on more than one occasion amounts to mental cruelty.

2. By addressing the chairman by name or the audience, as one moves to the final statement.

3. By a change in the tempo of delivery.

4. By enumerating the conclusions or giving a summary of all that has been said. And a good way to summarise is to answer A.B. Hill's four questions to writers of publications:

(a) What did you do?

(b) Why did you do it?

(c) What did you find?

(d) What does it mean?

5. By the use of an apt quotation.

6. 'So now you know what I think . . .'

7. The homily: 'I leave you with two thoughts: the first is that . . . the second . . .'

As with the introduction, there are many possible endings, but it is important to finish strongly. There should never be a need to say 'the end', 'thank-you', 'this is all I have to say'. The speaker should never wilt or fade away; he should try to work up to a climax, which will almost automatically invite a burst of spontaneous applause.

The conclusions should be so obvious that no statistics are necessary to convince the audience. Discovery, after all, is the art of stating the obvious first. Never show a table, graph or slide. Always be in full view of the audience with the lights on in the lecture hall: they want to see you at the finishing post!

In the final analysis, there are only three possible conclusions from the data you have presented:

● What everybody knows: even this may be important.

● What people thought likely, but unproven, yet your factual evidence supports it.

● What no-one had ever thought of before; lucky the lecturer who achieves that!

Even so, the lecturer will have to lead up to these three possibilities by describing:

1. his results compared with the theoretical,
2. results obtained by others,
3. reasons for any discrepancies or variations in his own data,
4. the efficiency of his apparatus or method of investigation,
5. the relevance of the methods used, human errors and any likely environmental factors.

He will also have to keep in mind what Mitchell calls the three-FYs:

1. simplify, by keeping to essentials,
2. justify, so that every statement is supported by facts and figures,
3. quantify, so that no generalisations are made without numerical support. It is for the audience to judge whether the lecturer has done so.

The advice of the King of Hearts (in Wonderland of course) was: 'Begin at the beginning and go on until you come to the end, then stop'. It still applies. The trouble is that some people don't know when to stop even when they have reached the end. The secret lies in anticipating the end so that stopping and ending are synchronous.

Reading or Speaking Freely

We assume that most lecturers will make an attempt to speak freely and avoid reading a lecture. However, there will be a few whose courage will fail them and they will carry to the dais a full script, in their trembling hands, to read to the cheated audience who assembled to hear a lecture and not a public reading. We also admitted in the introduction to this chapter that reading can be successful, but the script of such a lecture must be specially prepared. First, we shall argue the case for speaking freely, then we shall advise separately on how to prepare and practice a spoken and a read lecture.

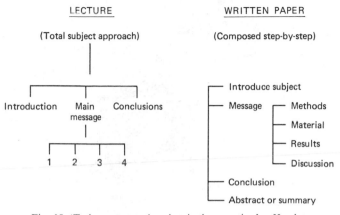

Fig. 18. 'To be or not to be: that is the question' – *Hamlet*.

● The Disadvantages of Reading

When talking the lecturer does not use a disembodied voice alone to communicate, but eyes, expressions, gestures and movement as well. A lecturer who reads discards all these.

1. He has his eyes downcast, instead of searching out and engaging the eyes of the audience.

2. His fixed expression is that of the frown of someone reading, but even if his face registers other emotions they will not be seen by the audience because his gaze is turned towards his paper.

3. His body is hidden behind the lectern, his hands used for turning the pages. Even when his arms flap feebly in a half-gesture it seems as if he only obeyed a written instruction.

4. He is tethered to his lectern and holds on to it grimly, like a ship-wrecked person to a raft. He dare not move to the blackboard, closer to the screen, or forward towards the audience.

5. Even his only channel of communication, his voice, loses its normal colour and vivacity to become monotonous and machine-like.

6. The lecturer who reads not only divests himself of most of his normal manner of expression, but also he deprives himself of his ability to receive messages.

In a spoken lecture, face-to-face with the members of the audience, one can react to their visible changes in mood; cut short a longish

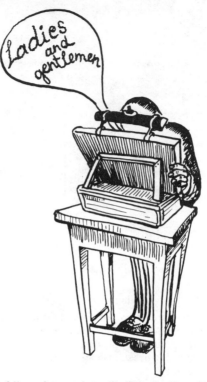

Fig. 19. 'A fellow of no mark nor likelihood' – *Henry IV, Part I.*

passage, change the tempo or introduce a diversion when the signs of boredom appear, or enlarge on a section which seems to arouse interest. This flexibility is lost when the lecture is read.

● **How to Read a Lecture**

A lot of people think that it takes less time and effort to write out a lecture and read it to the audience. So it does. For the man who says to himself: 'Sapristi, I've got to give a lecture next week,' it is the easy way out. But quite wrong. This lecturer is acting irresponsibly to himself, to his host, and to his audience: he deserves to be banned from the lecture theatre. No, there are no instant lectures, and few people have the panache to put over well a hurriedly compiled offering.

If you must read you must take this decision early. The preparations for reading a lecture differ from those for that which is freely spoken. Indeed, it may be said to be more demanding, as it requires a verbatim script. Also every sentence must be written down, with the knowledge that it will be read out aloud. The rules of spoken and written languages differ. The former relies on simpler words and basic grammar, it uses repetition and emphasis; while the latter is more complex, relatively rigid and formal. Writing intended to be read aloud must use short, emphatic sentences of transition and of relatively simple construction. The lecturer needs the skill of a playwright to write for a speech. He must rehearse it, reading it aloud to friends or into a tape recorder. He must alter and polish his writing until it sounds natural and flows easily.

When delivering the script, he must avoid all the inherent handicaps of reading. His eyes should not be cast down permanently; there should be pauses during which he scans the audience. Gestures and movements should be introduced and he should try to imitate, as much as possible, the actions of a proper lecturer. By taking a great deal of trouble and being aware of the pitfalls, a reading can be as lively and as successful as a spoken lecture. But we don't advise it.

Preparation and Delivery of the Spoken Lecture

Only the introduction and conclusion need be scripted. They should be written out in full and memorised. For the rest, the main headings or ideas only are jotted down. Each may be written as a brief note on a separate card. This allows freedom to rearrange the order in which the story unfolds. As with the short communication, practice and rehearsal should include, from the start, the use of intended illustrations.

The proportions of time spent in the presentation of various parts of a lecture compared with their preparation are vastly different. For instance:

	Delivery time	Preparation time
Introduction	20%	80%
Main message	75%	10% (because you know it and anyway that's why you were asked to speak).
Conclusion	5% (the conclusions should be self-evident)	10%

The paper for publication requires about 10 separate headings and the preparation time varies according to the complexity and detail required for each. Usually the 'results' demand detail and the 'discussion' a closely argued case. In a lecture both are out of place.

If the ideas are in logical order and there are good illustrations to sign-post the course of the lecture, there need be no fear of losing the thread of ideas in front of the audience. A temporary hesitation, while searching one's mind for the next sentence or for the best wording, will add rather than detract from the interest of a talk; these are the natural pauses of normal speech.

Pauses in the delivery are, as every actor knows, important. The first of these should occur at the very beginning of the lecture: facing bravely and scanning with his eyes the audience, the speaker should first wait a few seconds in complete silence.

It is extraordinary how electrifying this confrontation can be. The audience is hushed and waits expectantly. The lecturer, unshackled by the need of sticking to the lectern, moves slightly forward towards them and starts speaking. His voice should be loud enough as if addressing the back row, but his eyes should search out one by one the members of the audience. He is free to use not only his voice and eyes but also his arms for gestures and his body for movement.

Let us finish this description of the art of lecturing by quoting an artist (and a qaulified doctor), Anton Chekhov, in *A Dull Story*: 'I see a hundred and fifty faces before me, each one different from the others, three hundred eyes staring into my face. My aim is to conquer this many-headed Hydra. If at every moment I am lecturing, I have a clear conception of the degree of its attention and the measure of its comprehension, it is in my power . . . To lecture well, that is with profit to your listeners and without boring them, requires not talent alone but experience and skill; you must have a thorough grasp of your subject and be in absolute control of your own power and your audience'.

Hand-out

There are occasions where the lecturer will have to consider providing a summary of his lecture for the audience to read afterwards (some think it better to provide this beforehand: we don't, except for those brief summaries on research subjects where all speakers provide an outline as a kind of warning to the audience). The hand-out is useful for intensive courses, as a reminder of what the lecture was about, to provide references for further reading, to establish in writing those difficult formulae, as well as all that extra material which would only clutter the spoken lecture.

The hand-out should:

1. Give the title of the lecture, the date, the name and brief address of the lecturer (for those who wish to correspond).

2. Outline the topics in the order in which they were presented.

3. Use key-words to indicate ideas mentioned.

4. Be well-spaced out so that members of the audience can add their own notes.

5. Be prepared well in advance and revised critically before circulation: it is a cardinal fault to have to announce an error on the printed sheet.

6. Use A4 sheets, preferably duplicated from a stencil rather than photocopy paper which is difficult to write on.

4

THE SYMPOSIUM

'Scientific sessions are of secondary importance – meetings are for meeting people'.

Bela Schick

A symposium is a meeting at which several speakers talk on various aspects of the same subject, disclosing either different facets or a variety of views. The Concise Oxford Dictionary also defines it as 'a philosophical or other friendly discussion'! The word comes from Greek, meaning a drinking party.

The number of possible synonyms reflects the popularity of these meetings: conferences, colloquia, seminars and workshops. Whatever the actual title, they all need care in preparation. Full-time professional organisers arrange the large international meetings and there are more than five firms of conference consultants in the London telephone directory.

Choosing the Topic

The needs, the composition and the special interests of the audience must be kept in mind. In general, themes from the advancing edge of medicine are popular. In these fields books are likely to be out of date and publications lag behind research. Topics which concern research workers labouring in isolation or clinicians in new specialities may also be welcome. Postgraduate students preparing for examination will attend lectures on subjects which are poorly covered and difficult to learn from textbooks. Whatever the special interests of the audience they will all enjoy open discussion amongst expert contributors. Controversial issues should, therefore, be included and debated freely at symposia.

We believe that the symphony orchestra is the most wonderful device ever invented. Musicians of competence and ability play together in competition, as a team, with the discipline of self and the conductor; as a whole they are marvellous, as individuals worth much less. So too with a symposium. Speakers must know the 'score' before attending, and so speak to one theme although playing their separate parts. For the benefit of the audience there should be harmony and not discord.

Finding Speakers

The only way to find a good speaker is to hear him talk. Reputation in research, rank or status, are not guarantees for good lecturing. To invite speakers on the strength of their publications alone is positively dangerous; they may simply read what they have written and use the illustrations as slides.

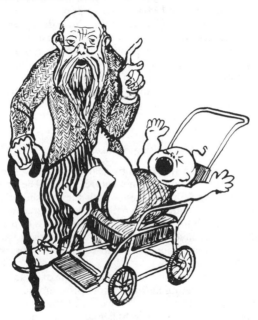

Fig. 20. 'Two stars keep not their motion in one sphere' – *Henry IV, Part I.*

Scientific meetings with a great number of short communications – such as the twice yearly Surgical Research Society meetings – are good forums to catch speakers. The fact that many of the contributors are relatively junior should not be a bar to invitation. Junior doctors regard it a great compliment to be asked to take part in a symposium and it is wise to mix people of varying seniority, to include the heads of departments with those who carry out the day-to-day work. They will bring freshness and enthusiasm to these meetings. Also junior speakers may be more amenable than their seniors to fit in with the overall plan of the organiser.

Famous names on the programme will undoubtedly help to attract an audience and a well-known authority is a great 'catch' for a symposium. Often these senior contributors are best employed as chairmen rather than as speakers.

The chairman should be allowed some say in the grouping of papers. To put three diverse subjects together and allow only one period for discussion is bad planning. The reluctant chairman may have to decide that the audience be allowed to discuss paper number one, then number two, a procedure which will inhibit the audience with different interests. The alternative, to allow free ranging questions, may lead to chaos or concentration on one paper only (to the annoyance of the other speakers); such an occasion needs skilful handling.

Several institutions keep a list of scientific and medical visitors to Britain (such as the Ciba Foundation, 1, Portland Place, London, W1N 4BN). These lists should be consulted and invitations sent well in advance to likely candidates.

Inviting Speakers

If the best way to find a speaker is by hearing him talk, then the best time to invite him is straight after his lecture. This will be a preliminary invitation expressing no more than a wish that he should come and take part in a planned symposium. After his verbal agreement a formal written invitation will follow. At this stage the details of the proposed symposium may not have crystallised, but as much of the programme as is already available should be disclosed. Further correspondence will inform the speaker about:

1. The agreed subject matter and the exact title of his talk, outlining the purpose of the meeting and the whole programme.

2. The time, date, duration and location of the lecture.

3. The facilities of the lecture hall must be described. To avoid repetition these could be given in printed or duplicated 'notes for the guidance of speakers'. They should include specifications of the projecting and loudspeaking facilities, details on how to operate microphones, pointers and lights, the availability of the projectionist (and how to contact him) and any special draw-backs of the lecture hall known to local speakers.

4. The speaker must be informed about the likely number, composition and special interests of his future audience. The possible presence of any experts or research workers in fields related to the subject should also be mentioned as a courtesy to the guest.

5. The amount of time available for questions afterwards.

6. The plan of the whole session must be outlined. The names of the chairman and of fellow-contributors should be given with their status,

special interests and the subject of their contributions. Speakers may also be advised to liaise with one another before the meeting to avoid overlap and repetition in their lectures.

The organiser must also fulfil his function as a host to his invited lecturers. He must offer help with travel arrangements and in finding suitable accommodation. He should inform them what the honorarium for the lecture will be and how much, if any, of the expenses may be paid by the host. He should draw his guest's attention to other events which may be going on in the same institution and mention any old friends or acquaintances of the lecturer, whom he may be able to meet on his visit.

On the day of the lecture, the car park attendant and the receptionist should be warned about the arrival of the lecturer and a special guide found to escort him to the lecture hall. All efforts should be made to smooth his way while waiting anxiously to give his lecture so that he will be treated as a welcome guest.

Advising Speakers

The foremost responsibility of an organiser or chairman is to ensure a high standard of lecturing and discussion. A careful choice of speakers will go a long way towards this, but some further tactful guidance to the speakers, on the form of their contribution, is also in order. To avoid trampling on sensitive toes, written instructions should be avoided; verbal and informal advice is preferable. A preliminary lunchtime meeting (lunch provided by the organiser or chairman!) may be used for tactful briefing. If time or distance does not allow this, the telephone is better than a letter. By whatever means, the following message must be conveyed to the speakers:

1. The time limit on their contribution will be kept and enforced without fail or favour.

2. They should attend the whole session, listen to other speakers, and be prepared to take part in the discussion.

3. They are expected to speak and not read.

4. They should use appropriate visual aids. If the contributors work in the same institution as the organiser then.

5. A rehearsal of the contribution, well before the date of the symposium, should be held, and

6. The preparation of visual aids supervised.

Some organisers ask for the script of a communication (for early publication) at the time of the lecture. The idea is to save time between the date of the symposium and the date of publication, which is admirable. But too often it is a useless exercise, because either the organiser will have a lecture script unsuitable for publication or a

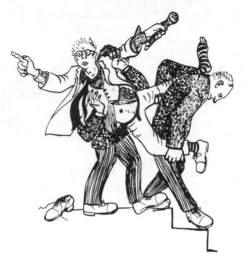

Fig. 21. 'Eating the bitter bread of banishment' – *Richard III*.

paper unsuitable for a lecture (back to a public reading again which will spoil the symposium utterly). It is rare to receive both, unless speakers are warned beforehand. Moreover the illustrations will (and should) be quite different for each medium.

The lecturers have therefore to decide on their particular topic, and then distil it: 70° proof is more likely to rock the audience than thin beer. Unfortunately, you can only distil, at best, three points to get them over; it is foolish to try for more. If there are other points burning inside you to tell the audience, there may be a chance to air them during discussion time. Be realistic, plan what you want to say, make sure that it will fit into the time available, and then translate ideas into easily understandable terms. On TV and radio, even difficult mathematical formulae and concepts are made easy to understand to the public by the use of analogy, anecdotes and simple language. The proficient lecturer has to do the same: do it well and he'll be asked to come again, do it badly and everyone will be pleased to see him go.

Administration of Meetings

A great deal of administrative work needs to be done for a symposium, but the details of this are outside the scope of this book. The interested reader is referred to a booklet entitled 'The Planning of International

Medical Meetings' (Paris, 1967) and Manten's (1976) book is another useful guide to be consulted. We shall give here a short list to check some of the necessary arrangements:

1. Advertising, the preliminary arrangements and method of enrolment.
2. Printing or duplicating programmes.
3. Booking lecture theatres, dining halls, meals, accommodation.
4. Preparing special route signs.
5. Arrangement for special transport.
6. Informing the supporting personnel: receptionist, caterer, projectionist.
7. Name badges, briefcases.
8. Communications with participants; facilities to call out members from the audience.
9. Social function, spouses' outings.
10. Finding possible sponsors.

This check list is, of necessity, sketchy and a whole chapter could be written on obtaining financial help alone. Pharmaceutical companies, for instance, are often willing to contribute to larger meetings in return for some sort of advertising – by providing labelled satchels, writing pads, and programmes.

Organisers should always hold a post-mortem after the symposium. Success or failure, it is valuable training to try to find out why. We have found questionnaires given to members to complete (but not to sign) to be singularly unhelpful.

Speaking Abroad

International medical meetings are on the increase. Many are little more than social occasions whereby one can meet people from other countries, renew old friendships and have a good time.

The man who lectures in a foreign land not only represents himself but also his countrymen. Those who are guilty of inadequate preparation denigrate themselves and their fellow doctors and, in our view, no-one has that right. To lecture well on foreign soil requires much hard thinking beforehand and a great deal of preparation for the unexpected. Even at large international meetings there may be no pointer and no silent method of signalling for the next slide; you may have to ask outright for your slide and this will interrupt the flow of speaking unless such has been practised beforehand. We record 12 items which experience has shown to be important for success.

1. If there is simultaneous translation then it is important to speak slowly, at about 80 words-a-minute. If you speak fast, the translator will omit some of your sentences and the sense of what you say may be

lost to the audience. Pauses in speaking are not just important, they are mandatory to allow the translator to catch up before you move on to another point.

A burst of speed occasionally is appreciated by those who understand your language, but not by the translator. Yet it is important to avoid a monotonous delivery because the interpreter will recognise inflections and variations of tone as indicating a change in the textual content of what you are saying.

2. Even quite long pauses will have to be interjected, especially before asking for the next slide. These are to allow the interpreter to catch up. He will be 2-5 seconds behind – perhaps 10 words, and may also be searching for the right word to translate your last remark. The easiest thing to do is to move back to the lectern while counting 1,2,3,4, before talking about the next slide, by taking time to put down the pointer, or by appearing to think what you will say next. The lecture can flow well, but a foreign audience will become confused if the translator is still talking about a previous slide when the next slide appears on the screen.

3. As much as we have condemned word slides we have to admit that they have a special place on this occasion. A few simple words on a slide can pull a lecture together; they should be pointers to what you are about to say and not complete sentences which would overload an otherwise valuable slide. Some lecturers prefer to have word slides in the language of the host country; this is a nice courtesy, but they must be translated accurately. A South American colleague will not provide Spanish suitable for Madrid, nor a Canadian the accurate translation into French for Paris. Word slides can also act as a sub-headings so that the audience may follow your lecture more closely.

4. Because of the inherent difficulties in translation from one language to another, simple conventional speech should be used, not a series of long words drummed up for the occasion. A lecture should begin well and end well and, again, never read your lecture even if others do so; it is better to be different and refreshing.

5. It is a good idea to follow up a point made by a previous speaker. By doing so you will help to fuse together a multilingual series of lectures and demonstrate that you were awake in spite of that look of concentration.

6. Good time-keeping is always appreciated, even if the other speakers show a complete disregard for the clock. The easiest way to overshoot your allotted time is to write a paper for publication and then read it aloud as a lecture.

7. Asking for the next slide may be a problem. If the projectionist is listening to the translation into his native tongue there will always be an interval of 2-5 seconds before the slide appears. Hence, our advice is

to slow down and to pause before requesting further illustrations. Alternatively, and this is what we recommend, you can learn some essential phrases (such as 'first slide, please', 'next slide', 'lights please') in the native tongue. But do practice the pronunciation and intonation until you have as near perfect an accent as possible before the day. The effort to learn even these few words and to pronounce them correctly will not be lost on your hosts. It's only good manners, evidence that you have taken trouble and have done some hard thinking beforehand.

8. Because slides may not appear immediately you demand them, it is imperative to rehearse several times with your own slides before your public appearance. In this way you will come to learn what to expect next and so can anticipate in words what will be seen. The advantage of slides containing simple reference points, such as 1,2,3, or A,B,C, can only be appreciated by a speaker who finds himself without a pointer and many yards from the screen.

9. Where distances of projection are great, poorly designed slides may be almost invisible if the ambient lighting is too great (which is common at international meetings to allow people to move around during the lectures). Whenever it is suspected that the lecture hall may be larger than usual or the quality of the projector sub-standard, we suggest that only black on white slides should be presented. Even then, the number of words and figures should be strictly limited. Eight to twelve words on a slide are probably enough and tables containing 3 lines and 2 columns must suffice.

10. In trimming down tables, particularly when a series is to be shown, one should be quite ruthless in removing unnecessary words and replacing repetitive words by symbols, such as +, -, 0. To repeat titles is wasting valuable space; it is even worse to include your own initials with the name of the institution and the date. Tables taken directly from previous publications are anathema; they contain too much detail which the audience cannot (or will not) absorb in the time available and to find 'Table IX' followed by 'Table I' is confusing, to say the least. Overcrowded tables need more than just trimming like an overgrown hedge; they require complete replanning.

11. In a large hall, the intensity of lights falls off inversely as the square of the distance of the projector from the screen. We all know this, but forget that the formula for comprehension is rather similar. The time (in seconds) for understanding what is presented visibly is equal to the number of words multiplied by the number of figures and again multiplied by a constant, K, which represents the complexity factor (on a scale of 1-10, according to the audience). Hence, 3 simple words and 9 single digits may take 27 seconds to absorb but, if the lecturer has not prepared his audience or has put his ideas over badly, the time may increase threefold so that even simple slides become

incomprehensible. The time allowed for a slide on the screen must be proportional to the information it supplies.

12. If slides are used to produce impact then a sense of realism should prevail. Forty-five words on a slide are impossible to read, so 100 makes the slide no worse. A reduction to 20 makes the content legible but 10 words or less will provide the impact required.

Films

Films are commonly used at international symposia (often without the author being present) even though they have certain specific disadvantages. Too often they are costly, over-long and out of date within a year or two of making. It is essential to have the correct projector and a skilled projectionist: 16 mm is the standard size film.

● **The 10 Advantages of Cine Film**

1. It alone can portray movement which creates reality. This applies to situations which are normally considered to be inert – such as anatomical dissections. Yet here the function of muscles can be shown convincingly.

2. The film can magnify moving structures which otherwise would be difficult to see or comprehend. Films of the middle ear, blood flow in capillary beds, movements of lymphatic vessels taken through an operating microscope all add a new understanding of these structures.

3. It can demonstrate a clinical procedure or surgical operation by altering the time intervals; thus a film can show all detail of the important part of a procedure at a leisurely rate, yet make closure of the skin incision appear to be completed in seconds (the reverse of the truth).

4. Diagrams can be interposed within the film for explanation and the salient features of X-rays, specimens and histological slides pointed out.

5. Difficult or abstract concepts can be illustrated and explained by the use of animation.

6. The film can be viewed over and over again until the observer is quite clear about its content.

7. Films made with sound may be a complete lecture in themselves and thus replace the lecturer. Many international scientific meetings have film sessions for just this purpose; they are usually very popular. The film can thus travel to a meeting without the lecturer and perhaps be almost as effective in passing on his message to others. But we don't like this method.

8. Time lapse cinematography condenses time and allows appreciation in a few minutes of movements that may have taken hours or days. Time can be slowed or speeded up, at will.

9. Short films, of perhaps 5-10 minutes duration, can be used effectively during a lecture to produce emphasis – by supplementing the visual experience and helping the visual imagination.

10. Finally, films can be made to allow the lecturer to talk continuously, with generous pauses for purely visual comprehension, without the interruption of slide changing or asking for 'the next slide'. In this way the undivided attention of the audience may be held.

● **The Disadvantages**

1. Films are usually quite costly.

2. They take a long time to prepare: it is best to allow at least 3 months to complete a 15 minute film, usually more.

3. They require special and costly equipment, a projector and projectionist (the do-it-yourself man fails).

4. They demand a great deal of extra effort from the lecturer. Effective film making requires a complete script which then has to be rearranged so that certain sequences can be shot on the same occasion (as in commercial productions). Much hard thinking is required so that the best use is made of the medium. The amateur's holiday film technique will not suffice, even with radical cutting and editing; some degree of professionalism is mandatory. In any case some experimentation will have to be done to decide when to use a long-shot, mid-shot or close-up, front view, side-view, above or below eye-level, to obtain the maximum impact.

In the end, of course, you may decide that a sequence of still pictures, shown as slides, would be better for your purpose; they are also cheaper and quicker to produce. Even when the film is completed, professional editing may still be advantageous however proud you may be of your gem.

TV and Teaching

There are other occasions when TV is thought to be the correct medium to use, often when your institute is 'in the money'. Such efforts are usually on video-tape, often in casette form. Before starting, it is worthwhile asking three important questions:

1. Is TV the most practical solution for what you want to do?
2. Will it save teaching time?
3. Will it save learning time?

TV is costly – in materials and time. To produce a good programme it is essential to be word perfect before any rehearsals begin (just like the professional actor) and to practise well beforehand all those expressions and right words that are important to your performance. Indeed, rehearsal in a studio is solely to acquaint you with the lay-out of the studio and the people who work there; it is not an opportunity to develop your own part in the programme.

The same effort required to make a film will be required from TV – the optimum viewpoint for the observer, the image magnification needed. Even if the script is not documented in great detail, there is still the need to be aware of what comes next. Unlike the conventional lecture, you cannot ask for the 'next slide' to put you back on course; you have to know and say what comes next so that the producer can follow you (he will provide the necessary, if only you will ask).

Ten Ways to Improve Your Lecture Performance

The more experienced the lecturer, the greater the risk of slap-dash preparation and presentation; such is nowhere more obvious than at a symposium devoted to the many facets of a single subject. Often the lecturer will have a well constructed and interesting contribution which he has given half-a-dozen times then surprisingly he is invited no more. What advice can one give to this speaker to help him brush up his technique? We would stress ten items:

1. **Be houseproud** by a tidy appearance, neat dress, standing up straight and never slouching. In other words, a good platform appearance. Slides should be cleaned, freshly spotted, numbered, faded ones replaced, and all presented to the projectionist in a good looking container in the correct order and the right way up for immediate projection (the spot at the top right hand corner).

Carry a new or well-kept briefcase (never a plastic carrier bag advertising a supermarket even though it may be conveniently to hand) to hold notes, slide folder, hand-outs and a collapsible pointer. A good salesman has a 'kit inspection' every day before he ventures on the road: so should the lecturer, and an occasional 'spring clean' to get rid of old material is always worthwhile.

2. **Be professional** by being an actor yet appearing natural: a touch of showmanship which doesn't show. Revise the text of a lecture by craftsmanship in sentence construction and be a wordsmith for the right term. This means writing a good script, which of course is never read to the audience and never presented exactly the same on a second occasion. Try to establish rapport with the audience early on by using appropriate gestures so that you get the 'feel' of the mood of your listeners. The professional always arrives early to survey the lecture theatre, to learn the names of people such as the chairman, his host, and the projectionist. The airline pilot always walks round his aeroplane and does his cockpit drill before taking off so that he can concentrate happily on flying. The lecturer should develop the same self-discipline so that he can make best use of the environment, the

occasion, or a chance remark to enhance his own lecture. The professional learns to think on his feet, to be prepared for mishaps, and to learn as much about the audience before it is his turn to speak. The professional has his own personal standards of excellence and keeps to them.

3. **Be observant** of new slide presentations, the way other people put over their lectures, new ideas, analyse what you see and hear so that these can be synthesised for your next lecture. Always be prepared to take advice when it is offered.

4. **Take trouble** to get the structure of the lecture right for that particular occasion and always get the facts right. Plan to interest and entertain that particular audience, which means taking the trouble to find out what the audience wants to hear and needs to know. Prepare and practice, well beforehand, what should be to you a new lecture and not that old tatty speech from a previous performance.

5. **Be courteous** by keeping strictly within the allotted time and keeping to the point. Do not make extravagant or unnecessary demands, nor make adverse comments on the facilities, quality and size of the audience. Never gossip about other lecturers, subjects or lecture theatres. Never criticise your host, chairman, or projectionist: they are invariably doing their best for you. Answer questions with courtesy, clarity and brevity. If the audience is unresponsive it is probably your fault, not theirs.

6. **Be obsessional** by being your own severest critic. Have a post-mortem after every lecture; write down the faults in your own performance, add a note on how they might be overcome, put this note with the lecture script and then file for future reference. Memory is fickle and only a written record will bring to mind all those improvements which can so easily be incorporated when asked to speak on the same subject again; by this means the second lecture will be different even if speaking to the second audience requires the addition to, subtraction from, or substitution of some of the original script. How can I do better next time? is the important question.

7. **Control** your own emotions of fear, anger or disappointment at all times; so smile and appear to be good-humoured, and let loose your imagination and enthusiasm for your subject.

8. **Pump energy** into every lecture. So, never finish feeling that you could have done better. Play to win and aim to be 'above average', which usually means that you will be drained of energy after the lecture and feel that you have no reserves left. Be dynamic in all that you say.

9. **Learn** to relax and not to be afraid to appear confident, but never over-confident. Learn to change your lecture technique to match the occasion; and never be afraid to experiment and learn to concentrate on your lecture while letting your eyes roam the room so that there will

71

be no 'blind' side (where the audience may begin to think that you don't know they are there). Learn to have an 'ear' for the reaction of the audience to your speech. Learn to laugh at yourself a lot.

10. **Appreciate** that your host has made all the arrangements to provide the lecture hall, facilities and audience just for you. All you have to do is to give your best lecture, because nothing less will do and if you don't you let down your host. Appreciate that every lecture is an act of salesmanship to sell new ideas and information to the audience. Appreciate that the audience will be on your side if only you provide a little encouragement. And be grateful.

5

CHAIRMANSHIP

'By God, Mr. Chairman, at this moment I am astonished at my own moderation'.

Lord Clive

When we go to a scientific meeting and people say that there was a good discussion, what they really mean is that everyone in the audience was given a chance to speak, a fair hearing, and that those lecturing were put on their mettle to explain.

The chairman's job is not just to keep order and be a timekeeper, but, like a football referee, to see fair play, make sure everyone has a chance to speak, make sure the questions are answered and that no one hogs the meeting. He should mention people by name which means he must ask first – this is not name-dropping but something more important. It keeps the meeting and discussion on a personal plane (one's own name is the most beautiful word in any language).

This does not mean that people should be discouraged from getting heated, far from it; every meeting requires some fire to wake up those who fall asleep so readily in the sitting position.

If there is any humour, and there should be because meetings are dull enough, then credit for this must benefit the speakers and not the chairman (he doesn't need public recognition, often he is well established or near retirement anyway). So no sniping by the chairman. But if a speaker has over-run his time and in discussion is asked a question then the chairman who interjects 'can you answer that in 30 seconds?' leaves an opportunity for the reply 'no, but in 20 seconds we have found . . . ' to get a laugh which he has earned.

So in a way the chairman sets up the situation and the important people, the lecturers, are presented in the best light with the greatest opportunity to shine. That is the chairman's job – an impressario, no more and no less. If he wants to be an actor then he should present a paper.

The functions of the organiser and the chairman overlap; indeed, at smaller meetings they may be one and the same person. There are, however, specific duties and privileges which concern the chairman only: the two should not be confused. The chairman has authority which must be unquestioned at every meeting; right or wrong in judgement, he is always right in decisions. He sets the tone of the meeting: hence the great value of humour, tact, a pleasing personality (and above all, authority) in making the audience feel at ease.

The chairman should define the purpose of the meeting. This may sound absurd when the advertised programme has already defined the purpose (such as for example: 'The place of antimitotic drugs in cancer chemotherapy.' 'Hypertension in young people') but even so, a short introduction stating the real object of the meeting is rarely amiss: it must be sharp pointed.

Before the Lectures

The chairman's introductory remarks should welcome the audience, introduce the speakers and the subject in a general way. This preamble should be brief, say 3 minutes, to warm the audience to the meeting.

He should call on the speakers by name and not just 'The next speaker will talk on . . .' He should not read out facts about a speaker – it looks discourteous. Nor should he poach the speaker's points. In a symposium, with many speakers, announcing the name and title of the next paper is enough but when the programme includes one or two lectures only, a longer introduction is customary. Here is an outline of such:

1. Speaker's name and subject;
2. where he comes from, his position and special interests;
3. the importance of the subject he will be speaking on; and finally,
4. a second mention of the speaker's name and a request to him to start his lecture.

If the speaker is personally known to the chairman this may be disclosed in the introduction. A short anecdotal story, if complimentary, may be used, but it is unwise to drag in a funny story to illuminate the subject. It may not strike the audience as funny, or the lecturer himself may want to use it. Above all the chairman should speak with respect and affection for the speaker, making him feel welcome and getting him off to a better start.

When introducing a single speaker at a major lecture the chairman has, on this occasion, the opportunity to talk in more detail. It should not be a mini-lecture but a few gracious remarks, to make the speaker at home and to inform the audience of the speaker's position, ability and his special qualifications to lecture on his subject (without actually discussing the subject). This may take perhaps two minutes: occasionally longer. But the chairman must remember that he is using up some of the lecturer's allocated time. Here are two examples. The first informs the audience about the elitist, but little known, James IV Association of Surgeons:

'On the night of 17th October 1957, three men sat drinking and scheming in Atlantic City. Two were Scots and probably sipping Glenfiddich, the third a New Yorker preferring Old Forest.

'The scheme was to establish a small select society of surgical leaders on the two sides of the Atlantic, to provide a bridge of knowledge, of research, of organisation and of education.

'One of the Scotsmen had just been made President of the Royal College of Surgeons of Edinburgh, to whom James IV of Scotland had given the first charter in 1505. And so the James IV Association of Surgeons was born. Ian Aird was the first President, John Bruce, Vice-president and Bill Hinton, Secretary. James IV was slaughtered at Flodden in 1513, but the Association lives on. In 21 years it has conferred distinguished membership on very few – about 200 – and from all countries of the world where surgical merit is recognised.

'I tell you all this so that you may welcome our distinguished visitor with due respect and some reverence. Dr. W. is not only a James IV Traveller, but also senior plastic surgeon at the University Hospital of . . . He is going to talk on some recent advances in cranio-facial surgery.' Then turning to the speaker, 'Dr. W. it is a privilege to welcome you' (start the clapping).

The second example highlights the personal relationship of the chairman with the speaker and relays this to the audience.

'It is a privilege to welcome you. We have never met before. But thirty years ago I followed in your footsteps. When you left the airfield at Scampton for the invasion of northern France, I took your place. You landed on the beach waving a mashie-niblick because, under the Geneva Convention, you thought a doctor should be unarmed. When I followed, I had a pistol but didn't know how to use it. From then on we continued our various ways. Thirty years later you have attained the highest position in the Royal Air Force (and congratulations on your recent appointment as Air Marshal), while I returned to University life. To-day it is my pleasure to introduce you and your subject of 'Major Air Disasters'. In my day, the major disasters were only two: running out of fuel and flak. We all would like to know how different things are today. Air Marshal X please tell us your views'. Then start clapping.

Apart from the introduction, the chairman should take care to acquaint each speaker with the local methods of signalling for slides, the lectern light, and where the pointer and torch rest. Some new modules are complicated (Warren, 1972), with more switches than a motor car.

During the Lectures

The chairman should show a personal interest in the lecture, he should look at the lecturer and make an occasional note. He has privileges during the lecture – he can interrupt a speaker for clarification, or to ask him to speak up or more slowly – in the interest of the audience.

The chairman, unfortunately for him because he may be blamed, is largely responsible for the poor quality of meetings. After all, he is in charge! As Williams points out, at meetings of the British Pharmacological Society chairman are empowered to tell the projectionist to remove illegible slides. If only more would do so!

At other meetings the chairman has had the courage to the embarrassment of the audience who felt the same way but did not know how to express their feelings, to stop a lecturer because he was 'waffling on'. It takes more than courage to stop a lecturer before his time – ruthlessness. But as Williams proposes, the comparative qualities of a good chairman can be stated very simply: tough, tougher, toughest. If he has warned every speaker well beforehand, then the audience who suffer should be entirely behind the chairman's action. 'We don't like to lose you but we think you ought to go': the refrain of an old-fashioned song which is still fresh.

He has, of course, the duty and the privilege to enforce the time limit, but he can also terminate the lecture or the whole session earlier than expected or extend the allotted time – after explaining his reasons for doing so.

In a symposium or research society meeting where there may be eight 10-minute papers with brief discussion between each during the morning, the chairman must not only be an accurate time-keeper, but use his authority to discipline those who do not conform. If he fails to enforce the time limit, the whole session runs over time. A single speaker can deprive others of their allocation.

The problem is: how can the chairman stop the inconsiderate speaker? It is wise to warn speakers at the start and to congratulate those who keep well within their time. The audience will appreciate that such discipline is for their benefit. Physical force should be avoided but there are at least seven ways of stopping a speaker:

1. The chairman can rise from his seat and stand beside the speaker to indicate that his time has run out. This gesture allows the speaker to give his concluding sentence without appearing harassed.

2. He can stand up and say: 'Thank you. Let's leave it there so that people can discuss your interesting findings.' He should not say: 'Belt up!'. That is offensive.

3. The use of an alarm clock is not advised by us: it has to be fairly noisy to have any effect (many speakers go deaf while lecturing) and this may frighten the audience.

4. A set of three lights on the lectern is commonly used: green while talking, amber at 1-2 minutes before time is up, and red to tell the speaker to stop. In theory this sounds fine, but in practice it commonly fails to have the slightest effect (which leads us to believe that speakers also become colour-blind during a lecture). The light bulbs are too

small and so flashing units (for the amber and red) have been introduced.

5. A recent addition has been to add a 100-watt bulb to the lectern set of lights. When this is switched on, say when the speaker has run 1-2 minutes over his time, the level of illumination is such that the speaker is almost blinded. If he is in the dark still showing slides at this moment, the effect is dramatic: the speaker stops, stunned. The chairman should immediately lead the clapping and thank the speaker.

6. The projectionist can be signalled to turn up the room lights at the appropriate time.

7. Finally, the chairman can allow the speaker to run over his time, and then forbid discussion to take place. Unfortunately this penalises the audience too, and is only possible when there is discussion time planned between each paper.

After the Lectures

The Chairman should have a couple of questions himself to ask and in this way lead the discussion and set the pace. But he must judge the mood of the audience. If it is apparent that many people wish to ask questions then he should hold his own questions until the discussion slows down, even discard them if the audience join in briskly and clearly are enjoying themselves. It is the chairman's duty to start the discussion by asking those silly questions of explanation, of detail, or of reasoning, which no-one else dare ask – yet many would wish to. If there is a known authority on the subject of the lecture in the audience, he will ask him to contribute; he will have asked permission first, of course, and not just single the man out by name and without warning.

It is also the chairman's task to limit the number wishing to speak during discussion time to those who make positive contributions; hence, unhelpful and unproductive remarks have to be cut short while constructive criticism is encouraged. It is not easy, but then nor is the chairman's job. It is the chairman's job to make sure that discussion keeps to the point. He must not allow irrelevant argument to develop; if he fails he will forfeit control of the meeting and the audience will lose interest.

Worthwhile discussion can only take place in an atmosphere of good humour. The chairman must prevent acrimony and bad temper developing, which is not the same as encouraging brisk discussion and repartee. A lot depends on the chairman's personality, temperament, and the tone he sets from the start. It is the chairman's duty to keep the meeting moving forward the whole time. He must therefore give those who wish to speak equal opportunity to do so – better still, allow people from different parts of the lecture hall to talk so that discussion does not become centred around one area only.

In the case of a dispute, the chairman must act fairly and impartially. He has to maintain proper order during discussion, and may insist that all remarks are addressed to the chair in order to exercise his authority; this is rarely required and may give the impression of ostentation. A most valuable function is for the chairman to summarise the sense of arguments for the benefit of the audience, when this appears necessary. He is as much responsible for the success and smooth running of a meeting as the speakers.

How to Ask Questions

Although this does not concern the chairman alone, some guidance on how questions should be asked and answered is pertinent here.

Questions are asked commonly for one of four reasons:

1. For explanation of a passage in a lecture.

'Did I understand you to say that . . . ', is a common opening sentence.

2. For information, that is, further detail of the subject. 'Can you tell us a little more about . . . ', would be a suitable beginning to the question.

3. For provocation of the lecturer, perhaps to make him defend some of the statements he has already made. 'You have said that thrombosis can be prevented, yet Smith showed in 1970 that it always occurred in patients with cancer. What do you say to that?'

4. To express a personal point of view or other and contradictory evidence. For instance, 'I must disagree with you about the late results of using vein grafts in arterial surgery. We have now 200 patients followed for five years with only a 2% failure rate.' This may not appear to be a question as stated but is usually interpreted by the inexperienced lecturer as one. A more subtle approach is the derisory, 'Do you really believe that . . . when recent work has shown . . .?'

In the political field, heckling by loaded questions (such as, 'When did you stop beating your wife?'), are common, but unusual at medical meetings. More likely is the questioner who has to speak to let others know that he is in the audience. A question which is virtually a second lecture need not be answered, in our opinion. To ask the right question is as much a test of critical ability as to give the right answer.

There are two virtues in asking questions:

1. Clarity. It should be clear to the lecturer and to the audience, exactly what you wish to know. If there are essentially two or more queries, do not place them all in one sentence. Rather, start by saying 'I would like to ask 3 questions. The first is . . . ? the second . . . ? and the

third . . . ?'. Then sit down and wait for the reply. It is often helpful to have made a note of each during the lecture so that if the lecturer cannot remember the third question, when he has already replied to two of them, you can immediately remind him of its content.

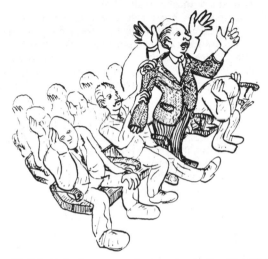

Fig. 22. 'Methinks I am a prophet new inspired' – *Richard II*.

2. Brevity. A brief question does not necessarily imply a brief answer, but usually it does infer that you have thought out the question before asking it. Brevity is good manners to others in the audience who may wish to place questions of their own, within the limited time available.

For the 'candidate speaker' – one who can speak well but has no lecture to give, poor fellow – this is his chance: he can go to lectures and ask questions. He can also comment and may even be asked to come down to the floor to say his piece. For him, better advice is to publish a paper on an interesting topic because then he will be flooded with requests to talk; when that happens, he can choose the subject of his choice which may be quite different from that of his publication.

How to Answer Questions

There are four golden rules:

1. Know your subject intimately: If you don't, you were silly to agree to lecture.

79

2. Hit back hard on tough questions. Go on the offensive when necessary.

3. Be alert and interesting all the time. Add humour to show your personality, to cool an angry situation, to score a point, and to curry the sympathy of the audience.

4. Argue like mad but don't give a second lecture. At the Royal Postgraduate Medical School, we put on three courses each year in specialist surgical subjects. More than half of the attenders are from abroad and they come for three reasons: to get up-to-date in their chosen subject (quicker and easier than reading the journals), to meet other surgeons with the same interest, and to hear experts argue as sheer entertainment. So argue.

Question time can be as testing as the lecture itself. The extent of the speaker's knowledge, the firmnesss of his convictions, his ability to stand up to a challenge or even irritation, will be tried and probed. A good impression left by the lecture may be abolished if feeble answers follow, but conversely, a lecturer who has read his paper stiffly may suddenly spring to life when replying 'spontaneously'.

It is worth preparing for questions. With some thought, one can guess in advance the most likely ones, and it may even be worth anticipating them by having a few additional slides ready. Also topics may be deliberately left out from the main body of the lecture in the hope of expanding on them (briefly!) in what will appear to be impromptu answers to questions.

There are nine silver rules worth remembering:

1. When he has finished speaking the lecturer should sit down, preferably in full view of the audience and look friendly and relaxed, to compose himself for question time. Jackie Stewart, on retiring as World Champion racing driver, advised the three C's for safe motoring: concentration on what you are doing, consideration for others, and confidence in your materials and yourself. This would also be our advice to the lecturer, about to enter the battle of debate by question and answer. He should also be alert to the kind of questions that may come and to the dangers ahead. Anticipation pays off.

2. He should listen intently to the questions, nod approvingly, and if there are several questions, make notes on a piece of paper.

3. He should never interrupt the questioner, even though he may think, after a few sentences, that he knows what is being asked. This is discourteous and the assumption may be wrong. If the acoustics are poor he should repeat the question before answering, for the benefit of the audience.

4. He should try to reply by using the questioner's name and look towards him, but aim the reply at the audience in general; so scan from side-to-side with your eyes and voice.

5. He should pay tribute to the question if it really deserves it.

6. He should keep to the point, be short but not abrupt. If the answer is likely to be long, or one which will not interest the rest of the audience, he should promise to discuss it further in private, or send details by post.

7. He should neither be aggressive nor personal in a reply. If he is provoked he may appeal to the chairman, whose duty it is to keep a sharp discussion within the bounds of civility.

8. Intellectual honesty is appreciated by the audience. If you don't know the answer to a question, then say 'I don't know', but do not then proceed to expand on your ignorance.

9. Do not be afraid to answer by one word: 'yes', or 'no'. You have saved time, have not prevaricated, and have given the opportunity to another person to put his question.

The chairman will observe the time limit on questions by calling out for, 'One final question, but it must be a brief one . . .'

Occasionally, it is best to finish early after a particularly successful or humorous answer, after which further discussion would appear an anticlimax.

Thanking the Speaker

This is the chairman's final formal duty and in some ways it mirrors the introduction. An important difference is that it cannot be prepared in advance. To be sincere it must emphasise some important quality of the lecture: its novelty of content, its polished delivery, or its entertainment value.

The vote of thanks should be short, gracious and dignified. The chairman may not agree with what the lecturer has said, indeed he may have questioned him in the discussion, but in his closing remarks he should not refer to disagreements. The closing remarks should be conciliatory if there has been an argument. Thanks should be sincere but not effusive. The chairman must remember that he is thanking the speaker (or speakers), on behalf of the audience; he should say so, and at the end of his vote of thanks, he should lead the applause decisively. Applause is music to the ear of a lecturer: it is the reward of a good performance.

On some ocassions the chairman may ask another person to wind-up the proceedings. This two-person management of a meeting is often appreciated by the audience, particularly if the second speaker has witty remarks to add.

The Special Qualities of a Chairman

A good chairman can make or mar a meeting just as a referee can a football match.

● He should be firm, warm and formal, but not officious.

● He should have a sense of humour: this is vital to avoid the inherent danger of his role – pomposity. At all times he must look happy.

● He should be impartial and should not try to hog the limelight: he should lead from behind not in front.

● He should have a personal interest in the topic of the lectures and in the lecturers.

● He should have complete control of his temper, have tact and be able to dispel any misunderstandings.

● The chairman may be more important than any speaker because he holds the meeting together. He should be able to stimulate the battle of debate, and know when to cut it short. He should encourage personal involvement and generate enthusiasm.

● He should have the experience and courage (often lacking) to ask speakers to speak up, to slow down, or to stop. Anticipation is the key to a good discussion.

● He should remember to thank the projectionist and any others who have contributed to the smooth running of the meeting, as well as thanking the lecturers.

● Finally, he should have a dramatic sense of the occasion and feel the atmosphere of the meeting. He can introduce a special kind of magic and fuse the whole meeting like no single speaker can.

In summary, the chairman should be like the gold setting of a jewel: he should provide the solid backing and embody the overall design, out of which the precious stones – the lecturers and the audience – should shine to their best advantage.

Listening

We add a note here about listening because to some extent it is more important to the chairman than anyone else.

Everybody hears, but how many listen? Listening is a very important part of communication because listening is conscious hearing. The main cause of faulty listening is loss of concentration by the hearer.

It is not easy to maintain concentration while listening: there are many distractions, such as extraneous noise, the movements of others . . . Thirty minutes is about the maximum time that a speaker can hold the undivided attention of the audience at a formal lecture: twenty minutes is enough for most of us, and the ten minute sermon is ample.

In effect, the concentration of the audience waxes and wanes at about ten minute intervals even with a good speaker and an interesting subject. Hence the skilled speaker intersperses his talk with a small diversion every now and then.

If we have little interest in the subject, we will not listen attentively unless we make a determined effort to maintain concentration.

• Barriers to Listening

1. Emotional disturbance. People with problems on their minds do not listen effectively. Hence many patients are unable to recall important detail of even the briefest consultation.

2. Dislike of the speaker. If we dislike the speaker (either from personal knowledge, reputation, appearance or accent) we tend to select what we want to hear; if we like a person we are more likely to accept what he says and to listen sympathetically.

3. Distractions are common at all lectures. The attentive listener concentrates that much harder to block out extraneous noises.

4. Tension. Listening is a positive activity and so a relaxed passive attitude is not conducive to listening.

5. Speech lag: The average talking speed is about 120 words per minute, slowing to 90 for special effect or emphasis; yet the average hearing speed is about 400 words per minute, which means that the listener's hearing has to slow down to keep pace with the speaker. This lag also applies to spoken words and written words: the eye can read much faster than the speaker can say the words – hence the absurdity of reading word-by-word from a projected slide: the audience will be way ahead of you. Here lies the difficulty for the active mind. What can the listener do about this speech lag to prevent his mind wandering and loss of concentration?

He can:

1. use the time to question mentally what has been said,

2. analyse the substance of the speech as it goes along,

3. anticipate what the speaker will say next and prepare his attitude to it,

4. dwell on points already said, but this is dangerous and may lose concentration.

Humour

Humour is the chairman's most valuable asset. Like bicarbonate of soda in a cake mix, it elevates a dull dish to haute cuisine, a mundane meeting to a memorable occasion. For the chairman, humour should be his stock in trade; with it he can rise above local squabbles, without it he may be in danger of being ignored. Indeed, we believe that a chairman without humour is naked.

We have tried to emphasise all through this book, that every lecture and demonstration has two main objectives – to entertain and to educate. This is the correct order of priorities: one without the other is an incomplete offering.

An entertainer needs a few props – a piece of chalk, a blackboard, a few slides, a tape-recorder, an overhead projector – for all have a place in presenting a live performance to interest the audience. There is, however, one ingredient missing – humour. Now, humour is difficult to write and is probably out of place in a scientific publication. In a lecture it has a special value, to drive home a point and to leaven the whole. Moreover, laughter will unite the audience, as well as holding their attention, because when we laugh we become a community. Sigmund Freud wrote a book on the subject which is well worth reading, if only to appreciate that a German joke is no laughing matter. Humour should not be dragged in, but flow spontaneously during speech so that it must be appropriate and pertinent to the subject. Some have intrinsic wit and for them pure sunshine highlights their remarks. The majority, the more serious minded, who cannot view everyday events with amusement will have to rely on jokes.

Jokes have a structure very similar to that of a lecture:

1. The introduction tells the listener of the situation and can be very brief, such as 'Two Scotsmen . . .'

2. The main part of the story develops the theme and builds up expectation. It is the serious portion.

3. The punch line is the funny part and, generally, the shorter this is the better.

Jokes also have rules – three do's and several don'ts, rather like life itself. The three positive affairs are:

1. Plagiarise; if you hear a good joke, jot it down and use it for the right occasion, but never disclose the source (unless the origin is particularly relevant to the lecture). There will always be someone in the audience who has heard it before, who will nudge his neighbour to tell him so; it is petty to deny that individual this small pleasure.

2. Always make the joke topical to the locality of the lecture so that the audience will realise that the lecturer at least knows where he is. For instance, if speaking in London, then, 'there were two surgeons who met outside the RCS in Lincoln's Inn Fields. The first said "I operated on Lord Smith last night for acute appendicitis". The second replied "Oh, and what was wrong with him?".' When in Edinburgh this should be changed to 'St. Andrew Square' and 'Lord Macintosh'.

3. Always rehearse jokes. The professional comedian rehearses intonation and pauses until he gets them right – so why not the amateur? More importantly the amateur should rehearse so that he tells the joke in the correct sequence; few jokes are funny if the punch-

line comes too soon. Worse still, the essential sentence may be forgotten or muffed, as in the story of the young vicar who opened his sermon by saying 'The happiest days of my life were spent in the arms of another man's wife – (a long pause) – my mother'. His bishop, present in church on the occasion, was so impressed that he decided to use the opening for one of his own sermons. But on the day, the bishop started 'The happiest days of my life were spent in the arms of another man's wife' and after a very long pause to the scandalised congregation, instead of the original punch-line, he ended weakly by saying 'and I can't remember who it was'. No doubt this raised laughter, but instead of laughing with the narrator, people laughed at him, which is quite different.

The negative advice runs thus:

1. Never laugh at your own jokes. They may not be as funny as you thought and, anyway, if they have been well rehearsed they will no longer be comical.

2. Never make jokes at international meetings, especially where simultaneous translation is being done. If the interpreter understands the joke he may be unable to continue; if he does not, then he is guaranteed to make the remark unintelligible in another language.

3. Never make jokes at the chairman's (or someone else's) expense even if you think the old fool should be tucked up in bed. This is discourteous and many a fine research project turned down for funds from a grant-giving body can be traced directly to such indiscretions.

4. Never make religious jokes for they too may give offence to the audience. Jokes about the IRA and Scottish Nationalists probably carry the risk of personal violence and so should be avoided. One might also add jokes about junior doctors, unless the lecturer actually enjoys being consulted at 02.00 hours for some trivial condition.

5. Never make dirty jokes because they too give offence. The audience will know better ones and there is usually a varied selection of such books at most railway stations for the bored traveller.

6. There are many admonitions which will come easily to mind. The last, perhaps the most important, advice is this: when humour is well received (and it's heady wine), never go on too long. If the audience want more, let them ask – but they rarely do. Laughter is sweet music to the ear of a lecturer, for it leavens the whole talk (like yeast in bread) and so makes your contribution more palatable. But it can be overdone. You are giving a lecture and not a variety club turn.

PART TWO
THE TECHNIQUES

6

LEARNING TO SPEAK WELL

'A good speaker is one who asks his critics and friends to tell him what was wrong with his presentation.'

Roy Meadow.

The voice is born of an impulse and a squeeze; a rather simple explanation, but it suffices. The impulse to speak sets the brain to work, ordering a sound. The muscles of the diaphragm and chest exert pressure on the lungs to send a stream of air up the trachea; this is just air, and, until it reaches the larynx, is soundless. The vocal cords vibrate to produce a musical note in the air which passes upwards into the pharynx to be amplified. The air stream is amplified again when it bounces off the elevated soft palate to take a right-angle turn to reach the mouth. The tongue, teeth and lips now form the sound into speech which is again bounced off the hard palate and projected into space. What could be simpler? Unfortunately not every structure is co-ordinated without practice, trial and error, and an awareness of how we want our speech to sound; pitch, tone, projection and speed are all under our conscious control. So we have to use them to best advantage.

The lecturer must achieve vocal proficiency because speaking is his medium of communication. This requires regular practice in the same way that a musician must practise before performing in public. The essentials for vocal proficiency are:
1. Clarity.
2. Words.
3. Rate of speaking, pauses and duration.
4. Rhythmic expressions, their phrasing and blending.
5. Pitch, tone and volume of the voice.
6. Emphasis, variety and animation.
7. Style.
8. Differences between written and spoken English.
Let us consider each of these in more detail.

I. Clarity

Clarity demands three things:
1. clear diction,
2. colloquial and familiar language, and
3. simplicity.

Clear diction is acquired by the correct articulation of the spoken sound and the pronunciation of every syllable. It is only possible to accomplish this by opening the mouth widely, with the head well up. At first this will feel artificial and forced, but learn to speak slowly in this way and soon it will become quite natural. In many languages it is the vowels which are important: in English, it is the consonants.

For those who are unable to master the art of speaking up, we strongly advise a little tuition, not speech therapy but some lessons in elocution. It is an extraordinary fact that boys at school are rarely taught to speak well, girls often. Parents seem to believe that investment in private elocution lessons enhances the prospects of a good marriage for the girl who speaks nicely. This may be true. But the muttering male would also benefit. While every actor spends much time and practice in learning voice projection, few lecturers ever consider that clear speech is the essential medium of communication for both.

Elocution lessons will not only improve the clarity of speaking, but also flatten out national and regional accents as well as giving a more cultured voice. This is not to say that doctors have uncultured voices (very few do), but many are sloppy in the way they normally speak and this will not do for a public lecture.

Richard Leech, a qualified doctor and actor, has written: 'I have been amazed to discover how few of the lecturers at these establishments (*centres of postgraduate learning*) have bothered to consider the basic principles of voice production and presentation: principles without which no actor would ever achieve his first job'.

Elocution lessons will make the speaker more confident, so that when lecturing he moves to the best position where there is good light and he can be seen by every member of the audience. The lecturer will move out from behind the lectern and not hide behind it, as so many do. As Leech points out, the centre of the stage is the best position from which to command an audience. A polished speaker does not drop his voice at the end of sentences, does not speak on the move, nor address the blackboard while drawing. He is aware of his audience all the time and speaks to them.

In normal conversation, a colloquial structure of sentences is used and these should be preserved in public speaking. Too many people who are clear and concise in every-day conversation lapse into tortuous verbosity in the lecture theatre. It is also wise to develop a feeling for the power and beauty of words and the gift of putting them together intelligently.

Simplicity in the construction of a sentence means using direct speech and familiar words. On the whole, short sentences are better than long, but variety is important too. Abstruse subjects are often made needlessly difficult and even the simple can be made to appear more complex by some.

Clarity is acquired by taking trouble and it is bad manners not to make your subject crystal clear to all; this can be done only by thinking and rethinking ideas and then by speaking to serve the audience so that you can be heard and never misunderstood.

II. Words

There is no law which says that you have to use big words when you talk. There are lots of small words, and good ones at that, which can be made to say the things you want to say; it takes more time to find them, but it's worth the search. Small words can be crisp, brief, terse, and get to the point; they have a charm of their own, they move with ease when big words stand still, they sing because you know exactly what they mean when you hear them. Small words can and do capture large thoughts, to hold them up for everyone to see. Small is beautiful in language.

The use of small words does not deny the speaker elegant variation, but the alternatives are often what Dr. Michael O'Donnell has called 'Decorated Municipal Gothic'. The simple statement becomes woolly. 'Go' and 'get' are surely better than 'proceed' and 'obtain'? Yet most prefer the latter, two more syllables to say and two more pebbles to confuse understanding.

Style is an important element in speaking, but is extremely difficult to define. It has to do with the way we use words, the variety of our vocabulary, the length and rhythm of our sentences, the use of gesture; it also depends on how we feel and who we are talking to. So style is largely a personal thing, like the way we walk and the way we eat. But it can be improved by practice, thought and care.

The choice of words influences style more than anything else, but this is governed by education, social environment, breadth of reading, understanding of the occasion and the circumstances of speaking. It has been estimated that the person of average education has a vocabulary of about 15,000 words which he understands, but uses only 3000. Indeed, in general conversation 80% of all that is spoken accounts for about 1000 words. A moderately sized dictionary will have definitions of a little over 60,000 words from which to choose, but they may not be understood by the recipient. In medicine, before he qualifies, a doctor has to learn the meaning of about 5000 words – more than enough for fluency in a foreign language. No wonder patients, friends and even colleagues fail to understand what we mean when we use these specialised terms.

91

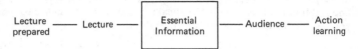

Fig. 23. 'Brevity is the soul of wit' – *Hamlet*.

Talleyrand is supposed to have said that speech was given to man to disguise his thoughts. It is clear that many lecturers think the same. But language is the most important means of communication, and words are the building blocks of language. Words are the tools we use in a lecture so they should be sharp-pointed. But speech derives meaning not merely from the words uttered. Words are coloured and amplified, sometimes reversed in meaning, by gesture, by variations in tone and volume of the voice, as well as by illustrations, analogies and questions.

As Mark Twain once wrote: the difference between the right word and the almost-right word is the difference between 'lightning' and 'lightning-bug'. In science, we can relate the difference as equal to that between cause and effect.

'Noise' in information theory is defined as any factor within or outside of a system of communication that alters the intended message (the thoughts the lecturer wishes to convey). All person-to-person communication systems suffer from interference from noise, but none so much as in writing or lecturing in medicine. Writing suffers because the English language is rather irrational and the writer and reader have no channel of feed-back between them. Speech suffers because we do not use the right word at the right time and commonly misinterpret the feed-back from the audience. The simplest oral communication system consists of a speaker, a message, and a listener. The speaker performs three tasks: he gathers information, encodes it into language symbols, and transmits these symbols as signals (words, pitch, tone, etc., plus gesture). The listener reverses the process: he receives the signals, decodes them into symbols and finally interprets these symbols as information which he then evaluates.

To encode a message in speech, the originator translates his thoughts into word signals and assembles them into units of phrases, sentences and paragraphs for his message. For success, he has to select signals that the listener will retranslate into the original thoughts;

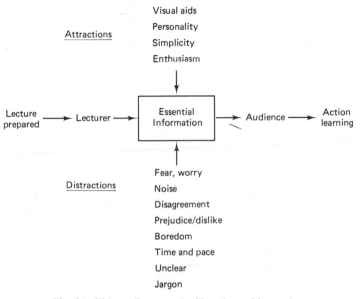

Fig. 24. 'Bid me discourse, I will enchant thine ear' –
Venus and Adonis.

failure results in semantic 'noise' and incorrect interpretation by the
listener. For success the lecturer has to:

● Select the right word which will convey thought clearly, efficiently,
and accurately to the majority of the audience.

● Define the specialised word and particularly the context in which
you use it. For instance, does 'day-care' mean that a patient is looked
after for 24 hours (and hence remains in hospital overnight) or that the
patient stays for treatment only during the hours of daylight (say 9
a.m. to 5 p.m.)? The listener must know what you mean.

● Make the context clear. The word 'programme' has a completely
different meaning in computer work to that of its general use as a 'plan
of procedure'.

● Prefer the plain word. Plain words are known to more people (and
more quickly understood) than the ornate and formal – which is not to
say that the latter should be avoided when they provide variety or
aptness. If the plain word does the job well, then use it.

Why say . . . ?	*If you mean . . .*
utilize	use
terminate	end
optimum	best
magnitude	size
unique	uncommon
conjecture	guess
necessitate	need
fabricate	build
proceed	do
comprehensive	complete
procure	buy
terminate	end
commence	start

● Beware of the -wise and -ize suffixes: most are vogue words which quickly become ridiculous (such as: weatherwise, heartwise, health-wise, moneywise, functionalize, finalized, democratized – and a lot more heard in everyday speech).
● Prefer the single verb to the verb-noun combination because long verb phrases distract the listener from what is important and slow down his rate of comprehension. They also clutter sentences unnecessarily.

Why say this . . . ?	*When you could say this . . . ?*
to make a study of	to study
to arrive at an approximation as to how much	to estimate
to take into consideration	to consider
to provide some assistance for	to help
to have a particular preference for	to prefer
to conduct an investigation into	to investigate

● Eliminate roundabout expressions by getting rid of words that say things indirectly: avoid woolliness at all times.

Woolly and wordy	*Concise and clear*
due to the fact that/on account of	because

in the event of	if
a large number of	many
a great deal of	much
at the present time/	
at this moment in time	now
despite the fact that	although
for the purpose of	for
it is recommended that	should
it is apparent that	apparently
it can be shown by tests	tests show
in a very few cases	seldom
in the vicinity of	near
has a tendency to	tends to
take into consideration	consider
it will be noticed that	(omit entirely).

● Try to avoid American English, partly because it tends to be wordier (with too many prepositions) and therefore lacks clarity, partly because the audience may be unfamiliar with such words.
For instance:

American English	*British English*
meet up with	meet
this point in time	now
miss out on	miss
regular	normal
figure out	think
terminal	fatal
let up on	stop
lose out on	lose

Some words have quite different meanings for commonplace things on each side of the Atlantic Ocean, and have to be 'translated' according to the audience.

In the USA	*In the UK*
Suspenders	braces
braces	garters
elevator	lift
candy	sweets
sidewalk	pavement
gasoline	petrol

- Leave out cliches and hackneyed phrases,
    - —Leave no stone unturned (except in Urology)
    - —Explore every avenue
    - —Be made the recipient of
    - —Stands to reason
    - —The cup that cheers
    - —Leave severely alone
    - —More sinned against than sinning
    - —More in sorrow than anguish
    - —The psychological moment
    - —At this moment in time
    - —But that is another story
    - —I'll come to that in a minute (rarely true)
    Substitute 'virile English': there's plenty about!

- **Jargon**

Somerset Maughan wrote: 'On taking thought it seemed to me that I must aim at lucidity, simplicity and euphony. I have put these three in the order of importance I assigned to them'. We entirely agree. What is correct for a distinguished writer is good enough for the every-day speaker. The use of jargon offends all three attributes. Moreover, as Pickering (1966) has stated, jargon imposes deception: on the speaker, who attempts to clothe a simple idea in strange language to try to magnify its importance: On the audience, who may accept a neologism as evidence of their own ignorance. To say 'The drug induced natruiresis and kaluresis' may appear to be succinct, but why not say 'The drug increased the excretion, in the urine, of sodium and potassium', if that is what you mean. The function of language is to convey information accurately from one mind to another and this kind of medical jargon inhibits that transfer, and some are deliberately coined to confuse. Ultimately, of course, jargon induces self-deception in the speaker too.

Unnecessary and undesirable technical jargon is one of the bad habits of our time. Not only do the words confuse the listener, most of them sound ugly. For instance, try pronouncing some of the new words (allergology, centrencephalic, hypohyperparathyroidism, pathophysiology, dysraphicus, cholangiolitis, cardiomyopathy) during a well-flowing lecture. Not only do they halt the lecturer in midstream, they slow down the understanding of the audience because the new words invented for etymological reasons are often inaccurate. So why do it? Jargon appeals to the illiterate, plain English to the wise.

What is jargon? The Concise Oxford Dictionary defines jargon as 'Unintelligible words, barbarous or debased language'. When one is told to avoid jargon in speaking, commonly the advice is to avoid a mode of communication full of unfamiliar terms. This is the nub. To a doctor, a technical report in engineering appears to be full of jargon; the reverse is also true. We have therefore to distinguish between 'gibberish' and a 'technical vocabulary'. Elder (1954) argued that if the technical vocabulary of a science is jargon than all such authors must be condemned, for in no other way can they achieve clarity and conciseness of expression in speaking. But what is the use of fine research if the results cannot be communicated to all who might benefit? Publication and reporting verbally are the end products of research, for without them research becomes sterile.

In medicine, technical terms have been defined and are recorded in special dictionaries. These words have been constructed and designed to serve the speaker's needs with precision and economy. Some words, of course, have different shades of meaning and, when used in statements, their precise meaning should be explained. This implies that simple words should be substituted for the technical term where possible; they should, as a courtesy to the listener, for the object is not to produce an orgy of difficult words for economy, but to speak clearly. Research has now become involved with 'management', where confused jargon is so common that one wonders how managers talk to each other.

Most of the new words are so joined together that the sense is always difficult to discover and often quite meaningless. This is a great pity because medicine needs a simple language, not a foreign tongue. If you really wish to confuse, then think of a three-figure number and string together the words corresponding to each digit in each of the three columns of the 'Jargon Chart' to produce the required phrase. For instance, 555, (synchronised incremental integration – or 'togetherness' in normal language) and 008 (overall management policy) are useful at conferences.

The Jargon Chart

0 overall	0 management	0 aversion
1 anticipated	1 logistical	1 expectation
2 systematised	2 reciprocal	2 capability
3 functional	3 transitional	3 flexibility
4 responsible	4 organisational	4 concept
5 synchronised	5 incremental	5 integration
6 projected	6 limited	6 implementation
7 balanced	7 marginal	7 ideology
8 compatible	8 material	8 policy
9 optimal	9 oriented	9 resources

● The Fog Index

Gunning, in his book *The Technique of Clear Writing*, describes the 'fog index', a standard towards which all authors should work in the effort to produce readable prose. The index is obtained by dividing the number of words in a passage, say a page of manuscript, by the number of sentences: then count the words of three syllables or more in 100 consecutive words, to give the percentage of words hard to understand quickly. The sum of these two factors multiplied by 0.4 is the 'fog index'. From his own research, Gunning found that an index of 12 was the danger level: above that, readibility was poor: below it, preferably at the 6-12 level, the script was easier to read. He also found that sentences containing on average 20 words or more made difficult reading.

The 'fog index' applies to speaking although we would put the level lower. For those who write the script for a lecture in full (which is good practice even for experienced speakers) the index takes only a few minutes to calculate. Sometimes the results are surprising. Medicine with its plethora of polysyllabic words falls too readily into the high index category. Yet it need not. There are shorter words, easier to say and quicker to understand, which can be substituted with a little thought for the listener. We suggest that a 'fog index' of 6 is the general level to aim at, the level at which a 12 year old can follow and understand what you say. Almost anyone can write short sentences even if it means only dividing one long sentence into two: most people can get rid of subordinate clauses, dangerous in writing and often fatal in speaking because the listener will rapidly lose the substance of what you say. Important statements should always be simple, clear and concise, but speaking continually in a telegraphic style is not appreciated; variety in the length of sentences is the key – some long, some short – but never unnecessarily complicated by long words. You may think that by using big words you sound knowledgeable: the audience may decide otherwise.

'Temporarily' has 5 syllables, and so qualifies for a word difficult to understand although commonly used in conversation and writing. Is there a way round it? Yes. You can substitute 'short-term', 'briefly', 'for the time being', 'instead of', depending on the context (and that is where *Roget's Thesaurus* helps). Flowing speech is just as important as the words you utter.

Pace (or Rate)

Pace (or rate) is important in speaking. The most dramatic statements, the lightest humour, the profoundest wit, the most illuminating revelations, will all fail to reach their mark if the proper pace has been misjudged. Pace is the rate at which the speaker presents information to the listener; not so much the speed of speaking but the way he times the important ideas he wants the audience to accept. The pace should be such that when the speaker presents his ideas the audience is ready for them and will give them full attention. Pace controls timing.

Three common faults are that:

1. Sentences are too long and too overcrowded with information. So, break up sentences into two parts and pause to give the listener time to organise his thoughts.

2. Speaking is too rapid, especially when giving numerical data or using technical words.

3. Some speak too slowly when there are no complicated ideas to put over.

Comprehension depends largely on the rate of delivery by the speaker. In general, most people talk too quickly. During conversation one may speak at 300 words-a-minute but the listener is being monitored continuously – the look in his eyes, the way he replies – so that if he does not appear to understand all that is being said, words and phrases can be repeated more slowly until he does. There is no such personal service available to the lecturer.

If you wish to know your rate of speaking, mark a passage in a book: count the number of words in say, three lines of print – to obtain the average number of words for one line – and then read aloud at different speeds 10, 15, and 20 lines against a stop watch.

It is advisable to speak at about 100 to 120 words-a-minute, on average, when delivering your lecture. This is a generally accepted speed for easy hearing and understanding. One should also vary the rate according to the content, to prevent monotony; for difficult data, speak more slowly. A rate of less than 80 words-a-minute sounds slow to the listener but can be used to good effect for emphasis. Bursts of speed are useful when complementing an illustration.

● **Pauses**

In writing, punctuation is necessary for comprehension. Thus, the full stop or period indicates the end of a sentence. The comma separates a word, phrase, or clause and so simplifies the meaning. The semi-colon breaks up a longer sentence into smaller sentences which may be linked by the similarity of the subject matter.

In speech all these are replaced by pauses of varying duration. We suggest that the comma be indicated by a break in speech of about one second; the semi-colon would require two and the period three seconds. Speech also allows a pause to be employed for emphasis. The paragraph is the unit of thought in a group of sentences in writing and its end in speaking can be signalled by a slightly longer pause of nearly four seconds. This duration of silence should be extended during the lecture when changing from one idea to another; it allows the audience to anticipate that a new step in the development of the subject has been reached.

● How to Change Pace

Often a speaker will say 'Now for a change of pace . . . ' when he really means that he is about to change the subject to something lighter or more serious. At the same time the speaker will usually change his technique of delivery. So how can a speaker change the pace of his lecture? There are at least 11 ways of doing so:

1. Change from statement to a question; and be sure to answer the question then or later.

2. Vary the length of sentences and pauses (paragraphs in written prose). A series of short sentences (fewer than 10 words) decelerates pace; over-crowding a long sentence will accelerate the pace.

3. Emphasize important material by isolating the specific statement with a pause before and after.

4. Use parallel thoughts in constructions: 'The engineer uses the same method to . . . '

5. Using visual aids: slides, the blackboard and exhibits, or use 'filler' slides to relieve the viewer of having to concentrate on screen and speech at the same time.

6. Use an analogy. One of our colleagues when confronted with an argument always replied by saying 'well, give me a for instance . . . '

7. Cut down on the amount of new or complex information being provided.

8. Modulate the speaking voice – quieter or louder.

9. Repeat statements or questions.

10. Regulate the choice of words, or question the meaning of statements already said (but this may put off possible discussion afterwards).

11. Summarise what has been said so far in deliberate terms.

● The Pacemaker

We all tend to adopt a basic pace in speaking according to circumstances. For instance, in conversation with friends about a limited subject we speak quickly; explaining to a patient what his treatment involves we vary the pace; talking to foreigners, we speak slowly and deliberately. As a general guide, we should consider four separate conditions at a lecture:

Condition	Subject Unfamiliar?	Subject Complex?	Pace
A	YES	YES	Begin slowly, continue at a slow pace.
B	YES	NO	Begin at slow pace, accelerate to normal pace.
C	NO	YES	Begin at normal pace, decelerate to slow.
D	NO	NO	Begin at rapid pace and maintain rapid pace.

Rhythmic Expression

Rhythm is the metrical flow of words and phrases and is determined by the various relations of long and short, accented and unaccented syllables. The term is also used to express the harmonious correlation of various parts of speech. Rhythmic expression, therefore, includes the wording, phrasing and diction of all that you say and in a well-constructed sentence the order of thought is never fortuitous. The vocabulary and rhythm of educated speech often make excellent prose; the reverse is also true, so that the reading of passages aloud is good practice.

Sentence rhythm comes with experience and usually develops in the natural order as one describes events from the general to the particular. Careful selection, to exclude unnecessary detail which will break a natural flow, is required; detail can, after all, be read and digested later from the published paper. Rhythm can be assisted by the use of alliteration, allusion, metaphor and simile. A sentence has to have balance in length, in the words used. If it sounds right when spoken, then it is probably right for the lecture. Euphony counts: we all like to hear pleasant sounds.

Pitch, Tone, Volume

There is a common misconception that to speak at a low pitch is a sign of emotional control and superior intelligence. This is open to question, but there is no doubt that such speech is difficult to hear. So speak at your normal pitch, but vary it for emphasis and interest; speaking at a high pitch is tiring for the speaker and for the audience,

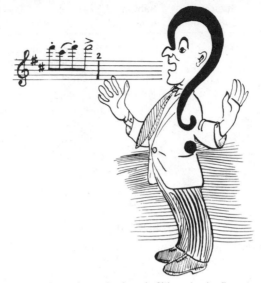

Fig. 25. 'He draweth out the thread of his verbosity finer than the staple of his argument' – *Love's Labour's Lost*.

but some accentuation will produce a sense of expectancy in your hearers. Thus when asking a question, rhetorical or otherwise, raise the pitch of your voice and introduce a note of query.

Tone is the quality of sound made in speaking, giving strength and colour to the voice. It is the modulation of the voice used to express vigour, emotion, and sentiment to the listener. It is also dependent on the connotation of the words used, which may evoke a favourable or unfavourable reaction in the audience: 'Village' and 'shanty town' both refer to small communities but the words provoke a quite different reaction in the listener.

Volume is the amount of sound emitted by the speaker and in a hall with poor acoustics the voice must be raised to be audible.

Emphasis, Variety, Animation

Emphasis, animation and vitality are personal attributes, but they make up for a great deal; to the man who really knows and loves his subject, these will come quite naturally. If you are excited and eager to share, others will warm to you: you become identified with the audience.

102

Inflection in the voice is a subtle method for producing emphasis and will alter the meaning of even a simple sentence. Consider the question 'does anyone try to prevent venous thrombosis?' which can be spoken in six different ways. Each carries a different meaning to the listener.

Does anyone try to prevent venous thrombosis?
– can it possibly be true?
Does *anyone* try to prevent venous thrombosis?
– surely no-one in the audience?
Does anyone *try* to prevent venous thrombosis?
– most of us do not try?
Does anyone try to *prevent* venous thrombosis?
– we are all more interested in treating it!
Does anyone try to prevent *venous* thrombosis?
– venous, and not arterial thrombosis.
Does anyone try to prevent venous *thrombosis?*
– thrombosis and not varicose veins?

Restatement is one of the simplest ways of achieving emphasis, but the key idea must be restated in different words to avoid monotonous repetition. It is, therefore, wise to build up a vocabulary of descriptive active verbs to improve the vigour and clarity of a sentence.

Variety is the spice of public speaking. One secret of good diction lies in the variety of words used, the length of sentences and pauses, and the rate of speaking; it is often the balance of patterns of sentences which carry conviction in speech. When reliving the scene and emotion of an anecdote, this comes naturally in the change of pace and pauses.

Animation refers to speech which has ardour, vivacity and is lively. Local dialects and phrases should be retained for they are part of the personality of the speaker. If these are more pronounced when you get excited, then get excited; the real enemy is dull lifeless speaking. The Scot's crispness, the Irish softness, the Welsh lilt, all animate speech. But, please, do not imitate accents and dialects that are not your own.

Gesture adds a new dimension to public speaking and is rarely overdone in the lecture theatre. Judicious use of gestures will animate the lecture because you will be acting the part too; in telling a story vividly one relives it with facial expressions and body movement – and these come quite naturally.

Style

Why bother about style? Well, what do you enjoy in a lecture? The content and the style are usually the most memorable. A lecture implies three things – a speaker, something to talk about and a listener;

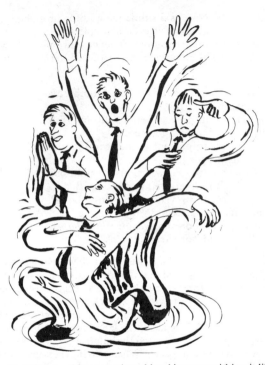

Fig. 26. 'Why should a man whose blood is warm within, sit like his grandsire cut in alabaster' – *The Merchant of Venice*.

the lecture unites all three but the manner in which this is done is the style.

We all have certain linguistic traits and expressive words which we employ in ordinary conversation. Jonathan Swift defined style as 'proper words in proper places' and the lecturer has to attempt just that. Voice and manner can convey important subtleties of meaning and evaluation, but it is the recognition of style which sharpens one's own expressions. The use of simple monosyllables with the occasional addition of highly connotative words, the organisation of sentence structure, the pauses between, all these form a personal pattern of speech. Style also depends on our way of thinking and of presenting data, yet the most elegant lecture is often the easiest to outline to others, which infers that style means clarity.

Differences Between Spoken and Written Language

English is two languages, spoken and written, and the difference between them is increasing all the time. The easiest way to appreciate this fact is to secrete a tape recorder when conversing with colleagues and later to read aloud a passage from a book. The former will immediately be recognised as spontaneous conversation, even though it may not make sense on 'playing back' (but it did at the time) and the latter sounds just what it is, a public reading.

These differences are shown by three examples:

Spoken	Written
'We'll get you in next week.'	'You will be admitted during the week beginning 12 August'.
'You've got the job.'	'You have been appointed to the post of Senior House Officer'.
'Your bowels are up the creek'.	'There are certain abnormalities in the function of your bowels'.

Here is a brief list of the main differences between spoken and written language.

Speaking	Writing
Grammar less obvious	Grammar important and may be either good/bad/correct/incorrect; word order gives the clue to meaning
Pauses not always equivalent to punctuation	Pauses are punctuation
Literal meaning can be reversed	Meaning of words is according to the dictionary
Sentences may be incomplete	Sentence must be complete units
No capitals in speech	Capitals start new sentences
Can point to illustrations and say 'look at that!'	Impossible in writing where 'see figure X' is correct form
Can use 'excess' illustrations to bring out opinions, ensure continuity of speech and allusions	Severely limited by editor; illustrations supplement or substitute for the written word

Humour valuable	Humour difficult and, in general frowned upon by editors
Alterations of pitch and tone can alert the audience to a change of subject	Impossible in written language
Pronunciation	Impossible in written form
Sounds can be used to good effect such as the voices of patients and music – and they can be dramatic	Irrelevant in writing and drama not welcomed
Personal pronouns used often	Rarely justified because medical writing tends to be impersonal
Meanings can be questioned	Not possible because confusing
Emphasis by repetition and accentuation	More difficult in writing, except by the use of italics or devious repetition
Word distinction is blurred unless context well established: 'The sun's rays meet' 'The sons raise meat'	Improbable in written language unless jargon introduced
Facial expression can convey disbelief, reverence, amazement, anger, grief	Much more cumbersome in written language

It should be noted that:

1. The spoken sentence is usually shorter than the written: gesture often replaces the need for words.

2. Speech is much less formal than writing.

3. The two forms are rarely interchangeable.

4. Written language when spoken sounds pompous, spoken language when written sounds brash and offensive.

5. The nuances of speech have to be spelt out in written language: the exact meaning of a spoken word can be reinforced by facial expression, gestures and voice inflection, whereas in writing it cannot. Even so, the exact word for the correct meaning you wish to convey is still important, if only to avoid misunderstanding.

The Special Value of a Lecture

The reasons for investigating some special aspect of medicine may be various – the desire for new knowledge, for the benefit of mankind, as a personal discipline, because of natural curiosity, or even for self-recognition. The end product, however, has to be passed on to someone else. There are two forms of communication; the written paper and the spoken lecture – they are quite different, although the object may be the same, to pass on information, and we have discussed that matter in some detail in the previous section.

COMMUNICATION

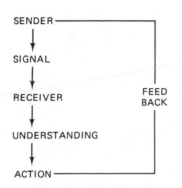

Fig. 27. 'She speaks, yet she says nothing' – *Romeo and Juliet.*

We live in an age where new knowledge is now pouring out at such a rate that journals can barely keep pace; indeed the information in a journal may be out of date before it is printed. There is, therefore, an urgent reason for the scientific lecture besides the traditional advantages of the spoken word. It is true that if one does not understand something during a lecture one cannot go back, as in a book – but such difficulties should be sorted out during the time for discussion and questions afterwards.

Lecturing is a difficult form of public speaking. To interest a passive and sometimes disinterested audience for 50 minutes is no mean feat. The lecture, however, does have special qualities which we wish to emphasise:

1. A lecture is analogous to a stage performance: there is no success without some training. The better the training the better the performance, if the script is good. Unfortunately, the lecturer has to write his own script and we have tried to show how this may be done.

2. It allows the speaker to bring out important differences between the lecturer's experience and what is recorded in text books. The

107

subject can be presented in better perspective, for it is possible to give alternative views and argue the case 'for' and 'against'.

3. The lecturer can stimulate interest and thought in a subject which may previously have been considered rather mundane. He can rouse enthusiasm in his listeners, which the written word cannot do. He can drive home a selected number of points which are well-defined, properly emphasised, arranged in the appropriate order and impart a better understanding or even a bit of philosophy, in a way that a book cannot.

4. The good lecturer can use visual aids to reinforce the spoken word and so leave a lasting image on his hearers. He can also show patients to make his subject come alive.

5. Listening to someone explain a new topic is often easier than sitting down with a book and trying to understand it. As we mentioned before, the special subject courses in Surgery at The Royal Post-graduate Medical School attract doctors to attend for this very reason.

6. It allows consultation with colleagues, for the lecturer to tell them what he has done and what he thinks his results mean. His listeners can indicate whether he should publish his work, do more, correct errors of thinking or technique. The object is to receive constructive criticism, and so the lecturer has to be sufficiently humble to accept what others say: he can argue his case, but in the end will have to compromise or admit to better ideas. If he will not accept advice freely given he had far better keep his mouth shut.

7. The lecture which interests colleagues should stimulate them and induce them to get up and put a contrary point of view, or even agreement.

8. It allows the speaker to put his ideas and results into final shape before submitting a paper for publication. The art of research is simple: be the first to state the obvious. Yet research is sterile without publication. We all agree that, because new data must be tested before it is accepted into the general body of scientific knowledge. That is what science is all about: building brick upon brick, from experience.

The published paper should give enough information for a competent and experienced person to:

1. assess the value of the observations,
2. repeat the experiments,
3. evaluate the intellectual process,
4. decide whether the author's conclusions are justified by the data presented.

But, if the ideas are truly new they are unlikely to be fully tested; they may not stand up to mundane criticism, they may need a lot of extra work for substantiation and the originator may not know how to proceed. The lecture, thus, can act as a sounding board for new ideas which have to be put over to the audience as 'new, true, important and comprehensible' (Lois DeBakey, 1976). Hence the lecturer may gain a great deal from the comments of his audience, particularly on items 1,3,4, when he discloses his data. In our view, details of methods should be reserved for the publication; even so, the lecturer will benefit from his peers by confirmation that his thinking is right, even though his methods may be wrong.

9. Finally, it allows the lecturer to answer those four questions, so important in research, posed by Bradford Hill in 1966;

> What did you do?
> Why did you do it?
> What did you find?
> What does it mean?

We have come away from many a lecture feeling cheated because one of these vital questions was left unanswered. We strongly adivse you never to leave the audience in that state.

The Good Lecture

The good lecture has seven special qualities for it must:
1. say something worth saying,
2. be free from verbosity,
3. make points with ease and directness,
4. be so phrased that it seems original and interesting throughout,
5. be stamped with the personality of the speaker,
6. have some parts which are memorable and quotable,
7. end in such a way that the audience are surprised by its brevity and wish to hear more.

At an international symposium you may be one of twenty speakers for a morning session. To stand out you have to shine. So keep to time, speak well, have no prompt cards if you dare, and be yourself. If you can also attain the ideals listed above, you will sparkle and be remembered.

Presentation

Mechanical noise assaults the listener from two sources – from the speaker himself and from the environment: all distract the audience. Most are preventable. The speaker may walk about with squeaky shoes, jangle coins in his pocket, fiddle with his glasses, ruffle his notes, wave the pointer, shuffle his feet, adjust his dress, wave his arms. Good advice: keep still.

The environment may be more difficult to control: such as noise from outside (loud conversation nearby, telephones ringing, building construction), whispering among the audience, interruptions by visitors, overcrowding in the lecture room, a noisy projector. The experienced lecturer will cease talking until some of this noise is eliminated.

Finally, simplicity. Although we spend most of our lives making complex problems into simple statements for the benefit of our patients, sometimes we deliberately do the opposite in a lecture. Too many speakers spend much time in complicating the simple when speaking in public and it is only during question time or in conversation afterwards that the difference becomes remarkably noticeable. The commonest 'complexity-maker' is in our own mouths: the way we use language and we have already commented on that.

We have said a great deal about preparation and practice for a successful lecture, but little about presentation. There are four aspects which require comment:

● Personal Appearance and Stance

Even before the lecturer has uttered a single word, the audience will have begun to size him up. For this reason alone it is essential to have a good platform presence with a well-mannered appearance. Dress should be neat and quiet, neither dowdy nor flashy and it is possible to be fashionable without being gaudy. A well-dressed speaker indicates self-respect and makes the audience feel that he is a dependable sort of person. Bulging pockets look clumsy and an open jacket untidy. One should stand up straight with the weight distributed evenly on both feet, which are set slightly apart to give the impression of relaxed authority. The object is to project your personality by appearing natural and friendly.

For the ladies, a new hair-do works wonders – they will put on a fresh face for a new day anyway – and feel more confident. The male will wear his best suit, perhaps have a special 'lecture tie' (one of us has: superstition of course, but no matter) and will look well-groomed.

● The Use of the Voice and Eyes

Where your eyes go, there will be your voice. Start by looking at the back of the room and raise your speaking voice a little so that you are loud enough to be heard at the back. Do not single out one individual for your whole attention: he will only feel embarrassed and begin to fidget. It is, however, wise to rest the eyes on one person in turn as though speaking to him alone; this helps to establish the idea that lecturing is organised, responsible conversation. Turn to all members of the audience so that you leave no 'blind side' in the room, for the aim is to interest the whole audience rather than to impress one individual.

110

Always start with a salutation, such as, 'Mr. Chairman, Ladies and Gentlemen'. This is not just good manners; it establishes personal contact with the whole audience and shows that you are aware of their presence. Such brief courtesy should never be omitted at the beginning of every lecture; you can say 'Fellow primates' if you must, but do greet the audience. In addition, if the chairman has made some gracious remarks about you by way of introduction, then remember to thank him at the start – you can even mention something about him, favourable of course – and such will please him and establish a relationship for all to hear. But, please, never be obsequious.

● **The Use of Gestures**

It is important not to pace up and down like a caged animal, for continual and repetitive movements are irritating to an audience. If you wear glasses these are part of your image – so do not fiddle with them – but one or two points in the lecture can be emphasised by taking them off.

Gestures can be used if they come naturally, although the actor rehearses these beforehand and the producer insists that they are expressive and appear natural. Some gestures that express various meanings are:

    (a) Open hands with palms up – appealing.
    (b) Pointing the index finger upwards and please not at the audience – emphasis.
    (c) Raising the shoulders – doubt.
    (d) Palms raised to head level to face the audience – reverence.

Many people wonder what to do with their hands. We believe that there is a choice, which does not exclude variations at different times during the lecture. One can hold the lectern firmly with both or let them hang by your side, but this looks stiff and unnatural. They can be clasped behind the back, which is popular with Royalty, or employed to hold prompt cards or notes in one hand at about waist level. Finally, one hand can be put in the jacket pocket, but not both in the trousers pockets which looks slovenly.

Some lecturers move about while speaking with the idea that it might be fatal to present a stationary target! Not so. If you have something worthwhile to say the audience will listen; if you don't they will not be impressed by movement. More importantly, when you move your shoes may squeak, the floor boards sigh, your lucky charm rattles – all to irritate the audience and distract them from what you say. So, please keep still.

● **The Lectern and Pointer**

The object is to be seen and to be heard, so choose your place of delivery with care. If the lectern is large, move away from it at the earliest opportunity. We have already suggested that the first few sentences of a lecture should be spoken standing directly in front of the audience so that rapport may be obtained at the outset. The pointer, or electric torch, should be held only when indicating a feature on the visual aid – (slide, blackboard, overhead projector), and put down quietly when not required.

The pointer in your hand is an inefficient instrument. It is often better to have an arrow on your slide and refer to that.

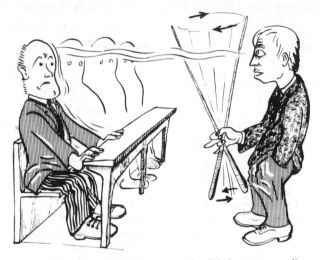

Fig. 28. 'He does it with a better grace, but I do it more natural' – *Twelfth Night*.

We would strongly advise speakers not to use a microphone unless absolutely necessary; it can only cause loss of personality and will not enhance it. Even with a microphone you will still have to speak up. The microphone does not improve your voice, it simply makes it louder. So, a dull, quiet, lifeless voice can now be more widely heard to lack expression. Moreover, the microphone picks up all sounds – bracelets, papers being handled, sniffing and coughing and even moving feet.

The best type is that worn round the neck for this allows the speaker to be heard when turning away from the audience. If there is a stand microphone, do not speak into it but towards it and do not touch it. The necklace microphone allows unlimited traverse of the head, but the stand allows only an arc of about 45°. In a large hall a microphone may be mandatory, but if the acoustics are fairly reasonable it is worth avoiding it altogether.

Finally, remember that most bad communications are due to defects in technique which can be remedied. Perfection in public speaking is an acquired attribute.

Prompt Cards

Noteless speakers are gifted rarities. You can become one with a lot of practice. Notes may be needed for a variety of reasons, but should not be literally read. It was Mark Twain who claimed that his best impromptu speeches were the ones he had most carefully rehearsed: we believe the same.

Notes are a courtesy to the audience, not a crib for the speaker. A sheaf of notes is depressing for the audience to see and hear, especially when written on thin paper. You can memorise your speech like poetry where every word counts, or you can just memorise the sequence of your facts and thoughts.

It is advisable to use index cards, 7 × 5cm, which are small enough to go into your pocket, and plain on both sides, but to write only on one side and to number them in sequence. The back of the cards can be used for notes from other speakers' material, for a record of questions asked and for that inspiring idea which comes to mind at the last moment. They should be held vertically in the palm of the hand so that they do not obtrude too obviously, or placed on the lectern so that they will not slip off. If held, they should be in full view at about waist level so that they can be consulted easily and, being stiff, they will not rattle when you place the top card at the bottom of the pack. There should be no furtive consultation with the cards which will only make the audience anxious. Consult the notes deliberately and openly, but try not to pause in your speech when the time comes; if you do, interest in what you have said will drop. Notes should be as brief as possible. It is wise to think over your lecture and your notes so that you are familiar with them and are sure that all the important points have been included.

Do not read from a flowing script: key sentences on a card are usually sufficient. If you wish to read an important paragraph, raise the card to an easily visible level to do so and deliberately put the card down when you have finished. Most people can read their own writing as easily as typescript and so it is worthwhile to make out your own prompt cards for you will be able to write at the bottom of the card and so economise in space, which the typist cannot. There is no limit to the number but we would advise 3 to 4 cards for one lecture; the intro-duction alone can be on the first card and the conclusion on the last.

You may think that you require several cards for a full length

INTRODUCTION

1. Importance to patient and surgeon

2. Mr. Jones – simple operation
   - good result – 8th May
   - pul. embolus – died

3. Treatment? Too late

4. Prevention – How?

5. Attempts in past?

NEW WORK

   - experimental
   - clinical trial

CLINICAL TRIAL

   - Randomisation
   - Type operation
   Diagnosis

RESULTS – slides

   - Age, Sex, etc.
   - Incidence
   - Treated Group
   Cancer

CONCLUSIONS – slide

1. Why bother? –
   –
   –

2. General principles (5) – slide

3. Planning – slide

4. Ask questions – relevant?
   – correct?

5. Selection patients (slide)
   – serial list
   – blind/double blind

6. Control group (slide)

7. Experimental designs (3) slide

8. Statistics

9. The Protocol (slide)

10. Getting started

11. Presentation of results

12. Conclusion: 10 golden rules

13. Examples – drug for D.V.T.
    – bleeding
    – antibiotics

14. Final conclusion: Progress

lecture, but, if it has been thought out and rehearsed adequately, two or three may well suffice. Finally, it is useful to remember that the prompt card system used for a 10-minute lecture may be applied effectively for an after-dinner speech. One of two cards, with larger lettering than usual can be rested on top of the brandy glass in front of you and so allay some of the nervousness intruding on an otherwise enjoyable occasion.

Opposite are two examples. The first two cards are for a 10-minute lecture on the prevention of venous thrombosis after surgical operations; the second two are for a 50-minute lecture on controlled clinical trials.

Copyright

Copyright is the right of property. In general if a work, whether published or spoken, is entitled to copyright it must be original. The originality relates to the expression of thought and not to the originality of ideas. The facts of a lecture are not copyright, only the way in which they are presented.

A lecturer may be able to show that there is copyright in his lecture, but only if it has been written down; it need not be fully scripted, a series of detailed written notes will do. Basically a lecture is a literary work and so should be protected by the laws of copyright in the same way that published diagrams, charts and photographs are. It is as well to remember that where slides are solely the work of an individual, they are protected by the laws of copyright. As far as we know such action has never been taken. We raise the subject here because in recent times bad habits (and bad manners for that matter) have been noticeable at international meetings. We deplore them.

Firstly, at many meetings someone in the audience will have a tape-recorder in use and a camera to copy the lecturer's slides. It seems certain that the recorded lecture and the photographs are, at a later date, circulated widely to those who did not attend the meeting, which is an infringement of a gentlemanly code of conduct and of copyright. Chairmen at meetings, in our view, should tell the audience of the legal implications of such behaviour which is also distracting to others.

Secondly, when a slide is made from a publication the author should be acknowledged on the slide (name, initials, date and abbreviated title of the Journal) even if the data have been modified. The recent habit of lecturers failing to acknowledge the work of others is bad.

The whole subject is currently being debated. Consult the detailed paper by C.H. Gibbs-Smith (Museums Association Information Sheet 9I.S. No.7 1974) published by the Museums Association, 87 Charlotte Street, London. WIP 2BX, and Flint's 'A User's Guide to Copyright' (1979).

7

VISUAL AIDS I – THE CHALKBOARD AND GENERAL PRINCIPLES, OVERHEAD PROJECTOR, EPIDIASCOPE

'Visual aids are aids for the student and not for the lecturer'
Ollerenshaw and Hansell

Discussion on visual aids is a popular pastime and deservedly so. Many papers appear with titles like 'Computer assisted evaluation of the effectiveness of closed-circuit television and tape-slide programmes in neurology', which to our minds deter further thought. Our concern here is modest by comparison. We would like to commend for a start the usefulness and the technique of drawing with a piece of chalk.

Drawing on the Chalkboard

In everyday teaching the easily available chalkboard has obvious advantages (Barabas, 1965,) but when speaking at formal medical meetings does it still have a place? We have recommended it at case demonstrations, at the 50-minute lecture and in discussions following a demonstration or a lecture, but we considered it unsuitable for the short, compressed scientific communication. We also believe that apart from specific occasions the blackboard (or as we prefer to call it, the chalkboard because not all boards are black) has a general function; it can teach the lecturer the principles of good illustration and the habit of 'do-it-yourself'.

The first principle of good illustration is that it should achieve complete accord with the spoken word. In chalkboard drawings this integration is almost automatic because it is forced upon the lecturer: he will have to go on explaining in words exactly what he is drawing with his chalk.

The second principle of good illustration is that it should use the minimum of detail necessary for comprehension. Again the nature of chalkboard drawing tends to ensure simplicity, because the lecturer has to memorise what he wants to draw. This usually persuades him to keep to essentials!

The third principle is the need for liveliness and nothing is more stimulating than a live performance. A chalk drawing takes shape in front of the audience; it may go wrong, it may succeed, but while it is being produced it is more interesting to watch than a completed drawing.

● Suggestions on Technique

Drawing on the chalkboard does not come naturally to the average lecturer, but with sufficient practice he can acquire the necessary skills.

Our twelve suggestions therefore are:

1. Practice drawing with chalk and learn the techniques before you use them at a lecture. The novice tends to hold the chalk too far away from the business end and often breaks it. Hold the chalk near its writing tip and learn to draw a firm line. For a broader line, as for shading, use the broadside of the broken-off piece. Keep the feet apart, and not together, so that the body weight can be shifted from one foot to the other as you write. In this way it is easy to write words along a straight line.

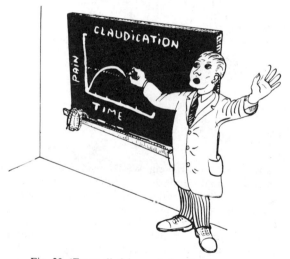

Fig. 29. 'Farewell, fair cruelty' – *Twelfth Night*.

2. Inspect your completed work from the end of the lecture hall for visibility and legibility. Acquire the habit of drawing and writing in large size, and so use the whole surface of the board. Apart from learning to handle chalk properly this increase in the scale of drawing and writing is the most specific problem in the use of a chalkboard.

3. Learn to draw without turning your back towards the audience, so stand sideways and from time to time face the audience.

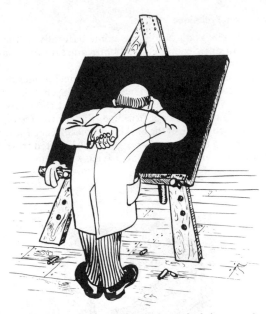

Fig. 30. 'If you have tears, prepare to shed them now' –
Julius Ceasar.

4. Speak while you are drawing. Whitwam (1970) wrote 'there is no point in spending valuable time drawing a diagram and then turning to the audience (now either restless or asleep) and presenting the completed drawing as if showing a slide'. Pitch your voice higher and louder while you draw.

5. Plan your lecture from the outset with illustrations. Start by drawing on pieces of paper while reciting the script of the lecture. In this way, the integration of verbal and visual components will be achieved early.

6. For complicated diagrams do not overload a single picture; rather use several sequential drawings of the same subject, adding different details in each diagram.

7. Many diagrams can be partly prepared beforehand by outlining them in chalk of a similar colour to that of the board (say purple chalk, or even pencil, on a blackboard), and completing them in white chalk in front of the audience, but they should not be displayed before you refer to them. (If there are sliding boards, a drawing on the posterior board may be hidden by the anterior one).

Complete the drawings in front of the audience by adding labels and important finishing lines. Erase a drawing once it has no relevance.

8. Tables and charts are extremely easy to draw but you must explain and label them. Allow time for the audience to assimilate and, if they wish, to copy them.

9. To illustrate special relationships do not try to produce a three-dimensional effect; use several drawings made from different angles. This is the simplest and least ambiguous method.

10. Use colour with purpose and the same colours consistently throughout the lecture, for example white (or black on a white board) always for lettering and for the abscissa and ordinate of graphs; red for important figures and, in anatomical drawings, for arteries or muscle; yellow for the same variable on different graphs or for illustrating nerves. Avoid colours which do not show well from a distance, such as deep blue and purple on a black ground.

11. Sometimes it is desirable to draw on the chalkboard during a lecture while slides are being shown in a darkened room. Usually there is a call for 'lights' so that the audience may see (always use white chalk on this occasion and write in very large letters), but this manoeuvre interrupts the flow of the talk and takes up valuable time. The alternative is to have an ultraviolet lamp focused on the blackboard during the lecture and to use fluorescent chalks. The result is extremely effective. Every item should be wiped off when no longer relevant because it will only distract the audience. The fluorescent chalks are not cheap and come in a range of colours: we have found yellow, red and green to be the best (available from The American Crayon Company, Sandusky, Ohio, New York, under the name of Prang Fluorescent Excello Squares). The UV light has to be of the correct wavelength (available from Theatre Project Services Limited, 10-16 Mercer Street, London W.C.2 – lamp No 230C and tripod stand) which provides a special blue-filtered light: the usual UV lamp sold for sun-tanning will not work.

12. Alternatively, the overhead projector can be used to 'over-ride' the lantern slide and a diagram drawn on clear acetate film shown; better still, use a separate screen for this.

● Chalkboard or Blackboard?

Seymour (1937) showed that a light-coloured board with dark lettering was more efficient than the familiar blackboard with white chalk. Both children and adults could read and copy from a light coloured board some 12% faster than from a blackboard. Hence, we have referred to a chalkboard instead of a blackboard all through this chapter. The best colour seems to be a light greyish-green. Some would even question the use of chalk, preferring the use of felt-tipped pencils. Unfortunately, to our knowledge manufacturers have not yet produced entirely satisfactory 'pencils'. The 'pencils' we have examined, contained coloured fluid which had a tendency to run out or to dry up, just in the middle of the lecture.

● The Advantages of a Chalkboard

To end our discussion on the chalkboard, we shall summarise its advantages in 10 points.

1. It is simple to use and inexpensive and, therefore, readily available. At the Royal Postgraduate Medical School, nearly every office contains a board – it's half the price of a projector and lasts longer.

2. It is most flexible in that diagrams can be altered and added to at will.

3. It involves the listener, because if the lecturer can draw a diagram so can he.

4. If the lecturer has taken the trouble to memorise a diagram, it must be important – hence, it induces emphasis.

5. It highlights the value of simple diagrams.

6. The lecturer remains the focus of attention and he is free to move and use gestures.

7. It is the simplest way of integrating words and pictures into a whole, to create the audio-visual effect.

8. The lecturer who uses chalk drawings frequently, will build up a mental store of simple diagrams for daily *ad hoc* teaching.

9. He will learn the principles of good illustration: usefulness, simplicity and liveliness.

10. He may acquire the habit of 'do-it-yourself' to produce other forms of illustration.

The Overhead Projector

The overhead projector is a natural successor to the chalkboard. Having said that, we must confess that we have not ourselves yet mastered the technique to our own satisfaction, nor have we come across a single medical lecturer who could use it well. Many lecturers still have a prejudice against it because they have only seen one of the early, imperfect prototypes. Improvements have taken place in recent years and in latest models faults have been eliminated. (For a full discussion on the overhead projector the reader is referred to Report No. 8 by the Experimental Development Unit of the National Committee for Audio-Visual Aids in Education).

This instrument was originally developed for classroom teaching in schools and any doctor who regularly talks to a small group of people –

such as weekly seminars or a regular course of systematic lectures – is well-advised to acquire an overhead projector and learn the necessary skills.

The Advantage of the Overhead Projector

1. The lecturer draws or writes while talking, so that all the dramatic values of chalkboard drawing are preserved. The projector requires transparent sheets of acetate film, usually 10×10 inches, on which words, numbers, and diagrams can be hand-written using spirit-based felt-tipped pens of various colours. Cleaned X-ray rilm is not as good as the special clear acetate: it is too blue, but in an emergency will serve.

2. The overhead projector has one big advantage over the chalkboard: the speaker faces the audience while writing.

3. There is no need for the room to be darkened (certainly with the new and more powerful instruments) so that the audience can continue to take notes.

4. No projectionist is required, as with slides and the epidiascope.

5. Diagrams and typed script can be prepared before showing: or half-completed diagrams displayed (to save time) and finished in front of the audience. The overhead projector, therefore, combines some of the advantages of the chalkboard with those of projected slides.

6. By using two or more sheets it is possible to build up a composite picture in front of the audience with telling effect. For this it is advisable to mount the acetate sheets in cardboard frames; these allow accurate superimposition by the locating notches in the frames, as well as making the sheets more durable and more easy to handle. The frames can be numbered in the correct order for viewing and carry titles for the convenience of the lecturer.

7. Moreover, by shifting one sheet slightly on the other, it is possible to produce the impression of movement in diagrams.

8. Alternatively all information can be produced on a roll of acetate, allowing the lecturer to move backwards to remind the audience of something he said earlier and forwards to continue the lecture. It is also possible to review earlier diagrams quickly, and thus summarise the lecture neatly.

9. Diagrams can be wiped off with 70% alcohol on a rag. Hence diagrams 'printed' in black can be used as outlines to which details are added or subtracted as required. Transparencies can be prepared without the aid of a medical artist or photographer, which makes it a 'do-it-yourself' instrument. With a suitable copier, printed material and illustrations from articles and books can also be converted to transparencies.

● The Disadvantages of the Overhead Projector

1. The instrument and the additional infra-red copying and duplicating machines are expensive; the office Xerox will copy well, but heat-resistant clear acetate film must be used.

2. The technique of using them must be learnt by the lecturer.

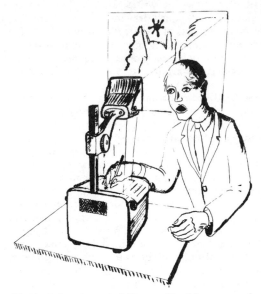

Fig. 31. 'And then it started like a guilty thing upon a fearful summons' – *Hamlet*.

3. For large audiences the projected image is not as sharp as from slides or a good epidiascope.

In his report on 'the overhead projector', Alan Vincent concluded that; 'no other teaching aid apart from the chalkboard makes such demands on the skill of the individual teacher, and at the same time no teaching aid offers greater opportunities to those who are prepared to make full use of it'.

● Overhead Projection of X-rays

There is no better way of demonstrating X-ray films to a large audience than on an overhead projector, but a powerful and specially designed instrument is required. The most important extra component is the set of folding shutters which can reduce illumination to only the relevant part of the projected film. In any hospital where regular case demonstrations are held, this instrument should be an essential part of the lecture hall fittings.

The Illuminated Board

This is a sheet of dense white plastic material on which you can write with water-base felt-tipped pens of various colours. We have been singularly unlucky with ours: the ink doesn't flow when required and wiping out with a damp cloth never quite clears the board. Moreover, there will be some who use spirit-based inks and these are difficult to remove. We do not recommend such boards but realise that they 'look modern' and are often installed by well-meaning architects (who do not have to use them) in new buildings.

The Epidiascope

We recommend the overhead projector for talks to small groups, but admitted that we have little personal experience in its use. On the other hand, we employ the epidiascope regularly at the Royal Postgraduate Medical School for:

    1. case demonstratons (in the 'Major Key')

    2. postmortem conferences, and

    3. rehearsals or informal presentation of short scientific papers and for lectures.

As with the overhead projector technical improvements have perfected the latest models and today's powerful epidiascopes are extremely versatile. They can project clearly:

    1. typed cards;

    2. pages and illustrations from journals and books, or photocopies of them;

    3. photographs;

    4. pages from case records and temperature charts.

● The advantages of the epidiascope are:

    1. its versatility;

    2. the lack of need for tedious preparation;

    3. much of the material projected does not require the help, in preparation, of the medical artist or of the photographer.

● The disadvantages are:

    1. a good instrument is very expensive and heavy,

    2. if it is not installed properly there is scattered light at the sides, which may be irritating and distracting for those sitting nearby,

3. the change from one illustration to another is not as smooth as with slides and takes longer,

4. a skilled projectionist is needed to operate the machine,

5. there is a tendency to talk to the screen (the OHP allows you to face the audience) and, as with the blackboard, turning your back on the audience is impolite. There are other difficulties; you cannot be heard (even if the acoustics are rated as marvellous), you lose your audience (because the back of the body is not expressive), and there is no feed-back to tell you of the audience's reaction (and they may have no understanding or little interest in what you have to say). So, remember please to turn to your listeners as often as you can. Never assume too much knowledge in the audience; dim-wits may attend your lecture, intellectuals too: both have to be catered for. The alternative which we recommend is to have the epidiascope cards photocopied so that they are in front of you and you can then face the audience while talking. Occasionally it is important to point to an item on the screen (which we advise just to add liveliness to the presentation) but on the whole data should be self-explanatory. By having photocopies in front of you, you can tell the audience quickly about the important facts while allowing them to read the list of normal results of investigations.

6. Epidiascope cards in a large lecture hall may not show up well. Hence it is important to check dimensions before deciding on this easy method of visual presentation. Enquire about the length of the room and the size of the screen. In any case, we recommend that Director type-face (IBM Machine) be used and that too much information should not be put on one card; it is advisable to keep the content small so that there is a state of expectancy (and not boredom) from the audience as the story unfolds. The standard epidiascope cards should always be used, if only to avoid a large hand appearing on the screen when each is changed.

• The Preparation of Epidiascope Cards for a Case Presentation

Special cards (28×16.5cm) with a ruled square on the right-hand side (15×15) should be used. The right way up is indicated above the square and the same design appears on the reverse side of the card. Only the area enclosed by the square is projected; the plain, left-hand side of the card facilitates handling and may be used for labelling with serial numbers. We prefer an electric typewriter for writing a short outline of the case history and findings on the cards. The letters will enlarge many times when projected on the screen and the slightest imperfection and the unevenness of ordinary typescript will look untidy. For the labelling of diagrams and for larger lettering dry transfer alphabets such as 'Letraset' may be used. It is important not to write too much on the cards. Only headings and signal words should be typed; full sentences are quite unnecessary. The lines should be well separated for legibility (double spacing on the typewriter) and there should be no more than 7 lines on a single card. It is preferable to use a large number of well laid out cards rather than to overcrowd a few.

Important results of investigation, significant facts such as the final diagnosis or findings at laparotomy, should always head a new card. If they are half-way down or at the bottom of the card, the audience will read them in advance of the story and their suprise value will be lost.

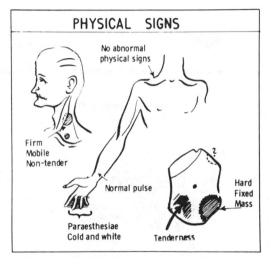

Fig. 32. 'More matter with less art' – *Hamlet*.

Many symptoms and all physical signs can be presented by suitable diagrams. The site of pain, the distribution of parasthesia, areas of altered percussion or auscultation can easily and simply be depicted in drawings. Temperature charts provide good visual summaries of the course of an illness to show alterations in the pulse rate, blood pressure and temperature, and their response to treatment.

Surgical operations should always be illustrated by drawings. As before, overcrowding is a danger and few operations can be clearly explained with the aid of less than 3 diagrams. For the diffident, body outlines either printed on a sheet or applied with a rubber stamp, may be employed.

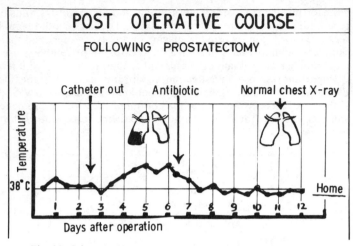

Fig. 33. 'Diseases desperately grown by desperate appliance are
relieved, or not at all' – *Hamlet*.

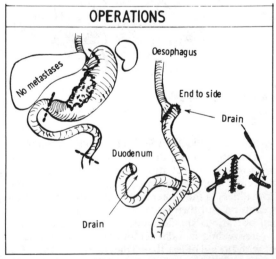

Fig. 34. 'We but teach bloody instructions, which being taught
return to plague the inventor' – *Macbeth*.

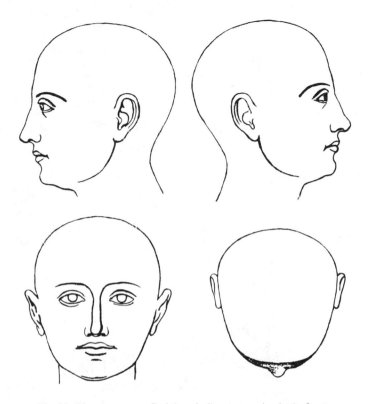

Fig. 35. 'There's no art to find the mind's construction in the face'
– *Macbeth.*

Relevant illustrations from books, journals, or case notes, can be projected by epidiascope. These should be photocopied first, the copies cut to shape and pasted onto the cards. In this way the relevant details only will be shown; any alterations or labelling can be added later. Furthermore, the handling of these illustrations will be made easier because instead of inserting books and articles into the epidiascope, the projectionist can simply continue with the pack of cards. The results of every relevant investigation should be typed on a separate line; abbreviations should not be used and normal values should always be given in brackets.

In the next chapter we shall discuss the principles of design for lantern slides. Some of these apply to epidiascope cards as well. In the

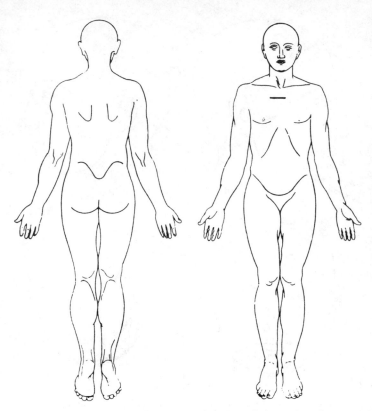

Fig. 36. 'In natures infinite book of secrecy a little can I read' –
Anthony and Cleopatra.

preliminary rehearsal for a lecture epidiascope cards rather than lantern slides are preferable and cheaper. These can be criticised by friends and colleagues and alterations made before the illustrations are finally photographed and prepared as slides.

8

VISUAL AIDS II – LANTERN SLIDES

'Lawyers with their constant opportunity for practice, show talent for public oratory that few doctors can equal, but the physician has one great advantage: he is allowed the use of slides'.

Zollinger and Howe

Of all the visual aids lantern slides are the most useful but also the most abused: they are truly weapons with a double edge. At an international congress in London, a distinguished doctor looked at his projected slide of a histological specimen, paused for a long time, and then said: 'I think that is upside down', as though it mattered! Well-designed and simple graphs can aid understanding enormously, but over-crowded, illegible tables may do the opposite. Good photographs may clarify a clinical problem, but poor quality snapshots do nothing but confuse and irritate. We shall try to advise the lecturer how to use this powerful weapon to his advantage.

Some people use slides just to be able to speak in the dark, having them changed at random, while not even looking up to see what is on the screen. This won't do. It is a gross misuse of a valuable tool. On the other hand, the lecturer with a complex plot and an intricate script will need excellent visual aids to put his message over. Whizzing through slides never compensates for rehearsal of a well-timed lecture.

Overall Plan

An overall plan of illustration should precede the design of individual slides. For a short scientific communication we advised slides to support every main point – except for the introduction and for the summary – like pillars supporting a bridge. The same plan may be adopted for a longer lecture, with the proviso that the audience should not be kept in the dark or semi-darkness for longer than 20 minutes.

Lantern slides should be planned to follow one another in an uninterrupted sequence; the switching on and off of the lights disconcerts the audience. This may pose a dilemma; what is the lecturer to do when he reaches a section unsuitable for visual representation? He can do one of three things:

1. Leave on the previous slide while talking about something else, or

2. Ask for lights, talk on without a slide, then have the lights off again and continue with the illustrations, or

3. Finally, and this is our advice, he can use a 'filler slide'.

Ollerenshaw (1962) recommended a plain neutral grey for this purpose but instead of an empty slide we would advocate one with a few words on it, summarising in a few short sentences the unillustrated part of the lecture. The background of the 'filler slide' should be light so that the lecturer may even step into the beam of the projector to be seen clearly during this mainly verbal interlude.

The steady flow of slides can be broken not only by actual gaps in the presentation, but also by illlustrations of strikingly different lay-out and design, A ragbag collection of photographs, mementos of previous communications, or even of slides borrowed from someone else, should only be used if the topic is anecdotal, such as, 'My twenty years in a rural hospital'. For most occasions a freshly prepared set of illustrations is needed. Special attention should be paid to the visual presentation of numerical data; if a graph is used first, it is unwise to change arbitrarily, for instance, to a column chart. The same design and the same labelling should be used for all related diagrams.

This care should extend to the choice of colouring. If the talk includes clinical photographs it is pleasing to have diagrams also in colour; if, on the other hand, X-rays form a major part then all other illustrations should also be black and white. Uniformity of design does not imply monotony. If several charts have to be presented, uniformity in their lay-out will help rapid orientation and understanding by the audience. The monoty of any presentation can be broken by including clinical photographs, sketches explaining the design of the experiment, or even a cartoon.

At the stage of general planning the first slide should receive particular attention for with it the lecturer may capture or lose his audience. The first slide should appeal to the whole of the audience, whose common general knowledge must never be over-estimated. The slide should be simple and general; a clinical photograph can be employed, for instance, when introducing a piece of purely laboratory research. The lecturer should remember that even when preparing for a moonshot the launching pad is at ground level.

Differences Between Book Illustrations and Slides

The lecturer must appreciate the fundamental differences between an illustration in a book and one shown on a screen; and the different effect of each on the viewer. Book illustrations and slides are not interchangeable offerings. We list the main differences between the two for comparison, so that you can see the advantages and disadvantages of each for the viewer:

Book	Slide
1. Distance to eyes about 30cm. Can be varied	1. Distance to eyes often 10 metres. Cannot be altered
2. Can use magnifying glass to examine details	2. Binoculars
3. Aimed at a single reader	3. Aimed at a large audience
4. Studied at leisure	4. Limited viewing time, usually less than two minutes
5. Reader can refer back to text for clarification	5. Viewer has to listen for explanation: if spoken words are not clear then the illustration is 'lost'
6. Can compare one illustration with another at leisure	6. No comparison allowed unless simultaneous projection
7. Usually complete commentary and legend included	7. Speaker has to unravel details and emphasise important points
8. Impossible to ask questions of clarification	8. Audience can ask for additional explanation

Why does a lecturer need slides?

This is an important question, not often asked because most lecturers expect to use slides and most audiences have come to accept them. But the question should be answered. A lecturer needs slides to:

1. Reinforce what he says: good.
2. Supplement what he says: that's good too.
3. Provide a visual memory: that is important.
4. Hold the attention of the audience: a poor reason.
5. Act as a 'prompt card' for himself: bad.
6. Show something unusual where description alone would be long, but visual impression quicker and thereby contribute to a better understanding of the lecture: excellent.
7. Complement his oratory: Oh, no.
8. Convey information rapidly: commendable.
9. Save time drawing on a blackboard and the need for 'lights': accepted.

Many lecturers abuse slides by:

1. Inaccuracies in spelling, for which the lecturer has to apologise to the audience (and so waste time for both).
2. Setting out data badly: it is easier to read from left to right and not vertically (unless you happen to be Chinese), but only if the lay-out is well planned.

3. Ignorance of the angle of vision, the laws of magnification, and legibility at a distance.

4. Overcrowding: don't try to impress the audience with the visual quantity of your data: tell them.

5. Useless punctuation: omit nearly all.

6. Failing to clean them beforehand: finger-prints impress no one.

7. Having too many.

8. Failing to look up at each when projected.

9. Using 'old' slides from a previous lecture: they have a faded look.

Principles

Now for some principles about slides and some simple arithmetic. Slides demand three attributes - visual, educational and time.

● Visual

Any photograph, drawing, graph, table, histogram, or a bundle of words must be immediately recognisable and understood by everyone in the audience. Please note that 'recognisable' and 'understood' are not synonymous. The slide therefore has to be seen clearly from all parts of the room. Admittedly a slide can provide a message in seconds, whereas speech will take minutes, but it will only do so if the visual requirement is good.

The visual component of a slide depends on the size of the artwork from which it was produced, the size of the lettering, the size of the projected slide (most lecturers use 35mm film, to provide a slide of $36 \times 24mm$), and lastly the viewing distance of the audience from the screen. It has been known for a long time that any object requires a viewing angle of between 10° and 40°. In other words, the man in the front row of the lecture theatre will have a viewing angle (or range) of 40° while the chap at the back (say 10 metres, or about 30 feet) will only have a 10° angle; at less than this he will need binoculars or see very little. From experience in designing cinemas, most architects plan modern lecture theatres correctly.

The viewing angle is calculated as equal to the height of the picture divided by the viewing distance. So, for the man in the front row who obtains a viewing angle of 40° this means a radian of 0.7. So, if X is the height of the slide on the screen in metres (we're Continental now) and Y is the viewing distance, then $0.7 = X/Y$. But we know from experience that X (the screen height) is commonly two metres (rarely more) so Y becomes about three metres which is the minimal distance for the front row viewer. For the back row viewer, who needs at least a 10° angle of viewing, the total distance should be no more than 10 metres, preferably less. All this means that there is a simple formula for acceptable viewing: the distance of the back row viewer must be less than six times the height of the projected picture. Hence, if you lecture away from home and bring your own portable screen do make sure that the seating is appropriate (take a tape measure for safety), so that your audience will be able to see what you want them to see.

Unfortunately the human eye can really only recognise two lines which subtend an angle of 1° or more so the person in the back row requires you to leave at least 3mm between the lines drawn on the artwork and between letters.

What has all this to do with slides? Quite a lot.

1. Capital and lower case letters should be at least 6mm high for easy reading.

2. All lettering should be more than 5%(one twentieth) of the height of the artwork. Hence, when labelling photographs or X-rays for reproduction as slides, measure the height because bold dry transfer letters will almost certainly be preferable to those of the typewriter. Try to choose the largest letters which do not offend artistically; similarly choose the lines for underlining data or division in tables (but see Reynolds and Simmonds 1981).

3. If you use an IBM typewriter with Director type face (for preference) you will have to confine the diagram and type within an area of less than the A4 international size paper of your typescript. Use an area of 14×21cm as maximum, but even this may be too large for good slides. Better still make a template from old X-ray film of 8×12cm within which the typist can work. For word slides, even this area is too large: confine such slides to within an area of 6×9cm – really quite small – and now you can use an ordinary desk typewriter (which we do not recommend) if you must.

4. It is easier to read data presented in a horizontal format, as opposed to a vertical one. So make graphs that way if you can.

5. Use the full width of the slide: the viewing angle worked out mathematically, depends on you doing so. Elimination of unnecessary data helps.

6. Sharp and accurate pictures are essential for good viewing. The artwork, the X-ray, and the clinical photograph (in focus) should be small before making a slide. When projected, the big screen will show your work to best advantage (and highlight poor technique!).

7. The height-width ratio of 35mm film (picture size of 36×24mm) is 3:2. The originals must comply with this ratio and, moreover, we emphasise again that every letter should be not less than a twentieth of the total height of the completed work: this constraint, commonly ignored, is more important than the information presented on the slide (see Reynolds and Simmonds, 1981, and Meyer-Hartwig *et al* 1977). Don't blame your secretary who typed the lettering for getting it wrong

(too small when projected): you did.

8. If data and drawings do not fit the criteria mentioned above then there is a choice: either stuff everything into one overcrowded slide and go through the detail of your figures one-by-one at your lecture (not recommended) or make two separate slides. Better still, leave out the non-informative data and explain why (strongly recommended).

9. Here is an extraordinary fact. Audiences can read, and can read faster than you can read aloud to them! So why read the words on your slide?

10. The Institute of Medical and Biological Illustration have published (Simmonds, 1980) guidelines for standards in designing charts and graphs. We commend them and look forward to further standards for illustration in general. Meantime, it is wise to follow Simmonds (1976) Rule of 4, which applies both for publications and for slides:-

A4 – maximum size for original drawing.

4.0mm – minimum capital letter height.

0.4mm – minimum letter thickness.

0.4mm – minimum line thickness.

4 units – maximum increment between thin and thick lines.

We would add that for word slides it is wise to limit the maximum to 4 words on a line and a total of 4 lines. On the whole, more than 20 words on a slide are difficult for the audience to take in quickly.

• Educational

The information on a slide either reinforces the words of the lecturer, or complements them. We have said that a lecturer, unlike the actor, has to write his own script. We now say that the lecturer has to compose his own slides for his lecture. Do not rely on the medical artist to design your slides: take advice by all means, but you, and only you, can provide the necessary data. Do not use slides copied from a publication: they look bad. You will have to bear in mind the answers to six questions:

1. How can I simplify the content so that all will understand?

2. How can I emphasise one point so that all may grasp it?

3. How can I make the slide immediately recognisable, especially to the one who attends after the lecture has begun?

4. How can I limit the number of words so that the man at the back can read them all in about 20 seconds.

5. What must I put on a slide which I cannot provide by speaking alone?

6. What can I leave out?

• Time

Every slide deducts time from your lecture. The slide demands time for the audience to see, the brain to assimilate and interpret, and for the lecturer to explain. If a slide cannot be understood by the audience in four seconds it is probably a bad slide (Evans 1978). Good slides can be shown at the rate of one every 50 seconds: we do not recommend this rate of projection if only for the comfort of the projectionist.

The one feature which distinguishes the published paper from a lecture is time. The publication can be long or short; the reader can scan and come back, read slowly or quickly, read piecemeal or complete at will, or file it and read later. The lecture by contrast is a single offering given at a specified time, lasting for a finite period, and then it has gone. We have tried to indicate how the lecturer should plan to use his time to best advantage and now wish to suggest 'time equivalents'. In the same way that carbohydrate equivalents can be exchanged to make the life of the diabetic simpler (for instance one thin slice of bread can be exchanged for a cup of cornflakes: hence no weighing is needed), so too for the lecturer the following equivalents (of speaking time, slide time, comprehension time and safety time) are useful to remember:

For every 10 minutes of a lecture you can—

1. Speak at an average of 100 words per minute. The typescript of 20 lines with 10 words to a line must therefore be no longer than 5 pages. From this total you will have to deduct all the other specified times.

2. If slides are shown then deduct for each about 50 words from the typescript, because this will be the average number of words required to explain the content of each slide. In a 10-minute scientific communication we have suggested that the maximum number of slides which can be shown comfortably is only eight. Hence deduct 400 words from the typescript, (which now becomes about three pages: but some explanation will already be in the script, so you can safely add half to one page more). Thus the total script should not exceed 3 to 4 pages. Another formula has been suggested by Professor D.N. Baron: 'one minute for every 100 types words plus half-a-minute for every slide. One sheet of double-spaced typed script on A4 paper will use up about three minutes of speaking time'. Our arithmetic agrees rather well. For the ten-minute lecture, six slides and three pages of typescript are all that you need (and probably even this is more than required). In effect, the condensed, distilled, and tightly knit contribution is quite small: the emphasis must be on providing punch – make every word and every slide count.

3. If the lecture consisted entirely of slides the total number should rarely exceed 20, allowing only half-a-minute on average for each slide.

For the slide with complex data two minutes is a reasonable period for the audience to assimilate the content. Moreover, only two facts per slide can be taken in, more cannot: it is safer to try to keep to one fact, one point, for each slide.

4. It takes the average audience about two minutes to digest a new concept, hypothesis, or proposition when presented clearly by the speaker; hence only three ideas at most can go into the ten-minute lecture.

5. Deduct 30 seconds for a slow start and a further 30 seconds for misjudgement of pace, a total of one minute which makes sure that you keep within your alloted lecture time. This means that you may have to delete a further 50-100 words from the script or omit one slide. The speaker who goes beyond his allotted time is not just a bad planner: he shows himself to be incompetent, ill-mannered and conceited. He may also make the audience hostile. Yet, a thought; no one has ever been blamed for failing to use all of his time

The Individual Slides and Their Design

1. Word Slides

Fashion also affects medical meetings and the recent vogue for projecting whole sentences on the screen and reading them aloud is deplorable. (There is only one thing worse than reading the script on the slide aloud, and that is to point to each word as you do so). Verbal slides are at best a compromise between having no visual aids at all and having suitable ones; they more often detract from, rather than aid, comprehension.

Perhaps this is putting it too strongly for we have to admit that there are exceptions. One good compromise is the 'filler slide'; another is for quotations which are humourous or particularly apt to illuminate one's own topic, and these are best reserved for the introduction or for the conclusion. The speaker need not read them.

Long verbal slides to summarise conclusions should be avoided. Reading them is tedious and they produce an anticlimax just when a final lift of interest is needed. Slides for conclusions, just like those for the introduction should be interesting, simple and visual; alternatively, one can speak slowly and emphatically, without visual aids and with the room lights on.

Word slides do have one important place – that is when lecturing in a foreign country. A few words can act as sub-headings so that the audience may follow you more closely. Do not read them out and do allow time for the audience to read.

If simultaneous projection is available then a word slide on the left of the screen complements the specimen on the right. This technique requires careful preparation and practice so that both slides are always changed at the same time. Never try to hold one slide back: always have a replicate slide.

2. Tables

Strong words are needed to condemn bad tables; often they are not visual aids at all, but instruments of torture. Some data can be given in none other than tabular form, but before the lecturer accepts this a conscientious search should always be made for an alternative presentation. If everything else fails, and as a last resort, tables may be used but strict and dogmatic rules must be observed.

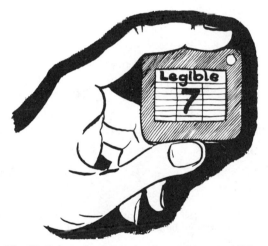

Fig. 37. 'It is a wise father that knows his own child' –
The Merchant of Venice.

● *Rules for tables*

1. Never use more than seven lines and three columns in any table and we believe this is too much, even for an intelligent audience and a slick lecturer. The seven lines should include the title of the table and any important footnote. If you think your data cannot be fitted into such a small table then look for subdivisions in the results, and prepare a separate table for each unit. It is essential to pre-digest and edit all results before presenting them in a lecture. Data which require long complicated tables to describe are not suitable for a lecture.

A

TABLE 10.

Electrolytes : 20 Greyhounds : means & standard Deviations (M.Eq./litre).

(all cages in situ for 3 – 6 months).

Electrolyte	Blood Serum	Tissue cage fluid	Significance of difference
Sodium	150.80 (2.61)	152.57 (3.94)	Nil
Potassium	4.70 (0.0276)	4.27 (0.0245)	P > 0.001
Chloride	106.97 (3.79)	118.27 (2.79)	P > 0.001
Urea	24.40 (5.51)	27.71 (5.94)	Nil

ELECTROLYTES

MEANS AND STANDARD DEVIATIONS

B

	Serum	Cage fluid	Significance
Na	151 (2.6)	153 (3.9)	–
K	4.7 (.03)	4.3 (.02)	P > .001
Cl	107 (3.8)	118 (2.8)	P > .001

Fig. 38. 'They are sick that surfeit with too much as they that starve with nothing' – *The Merchant of Venice*.

2. The writing should be easily legible by the naked eye when the slides are held in the hand at arm's length; if the script cannot be read in this way it may well be illegible on the screen. (Zollinger and Howe, 1964). Tables of data suitable for written publication (Fig. 38A) are highly unsuitable for a lecture and must be altered (Fig. 38B). Note the use of smaller type for standard deviations; even so, the slide could be improved by omitting them and by using lower case letters for the title.

3. Use the whole surface of the screen. Tables on slides need no drawn outer box, for the edge of the mount itself will provide the frame. If a separate box is drawn and photographed, valuable space is left empty on the screen when the slide is projected. Remember also that the transparent area is not square but oblong, measuring 36 x 24 millimetres; tables, therefore, should be designed to these proportions.

3. Graphs or Curve Charts

Graphs depict changes of one measurement against another and make good slides. We have seen some on the screen which must have been intended and designed for the printed page; graphs which can be studied at leisure while reading, should be totally different from those used in a lecture. For the latter, the principles are the same as for all slides:

1. They must be kept simple – one curve is enough and two curves should be regarded as the maximum. If there are more than two curves try to use two slides instead of overcrowding one.

2. Space should not be wasted, so choose scales for the abscissa and the ordinate to fill the viewing area of the transparency.

Use clear but minimal labelling; the judicious use of colour and good lettering is especially important for graphs and we shall deal with this later. In a monochrome slide, if more than one curve has to be plotted on a graph, broken and unbroken lines are employed instead of different colours.

4. Column and Bar Charts

Column and bar charts should illustrate comparisons. They are closely related, for a column chart becomes a bar chart when tilted 90°. However, a bar chart is preferable for at least two situations. The first is when durations of time are compared, such as the survival times (in years or months) following a particular diagnosis or operation. It is customary to express time horizontally, from left to right, and it would be confusing to show it vertically by a columnar chart. The second application is when the units to be compared need verbal labels of some length, as in the Department of Health circulars comparing the prices of various drugs. The labels are more easily placed and read one above another on the left-hand side of a bar chart than if placed beneath a column chart.

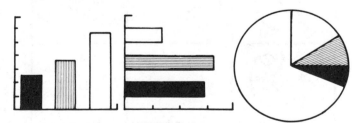

Fig. 39. 'An ill-favoured thing, Sir, but mine own' –
As You Like It.

139

5. Pie Charts

The pie chart is an attractive form of illustration with a rather specialised application. It is best for illustrating the division of a whole into parts like the slices of a pie, but the slices must not be too numerous not too small; three to five divisions are ideal.

6. Picture Charts and Combination Charts

When making comparisons, a drawing of the actual entities may replace the columns, bars or slices; for instance, soldiers standing on a map may represent, by their number or size, the strength of various armies. In medicine, the frequency of gall stones in various parts of the biliary system can be illustrated in this kind of so-called picture graph and there are several other instances where the method applies.

In a combination chart a small drawing or silhouette is used instead of written labels. Such visual vignettes can be comprehended more quickly and easily than words. The use of small diagrams instead of lettering is shown in figure 40. The table illustrates the higher rate of amputation in patients with arteriosclerosis who also have a duodenal ulcer.

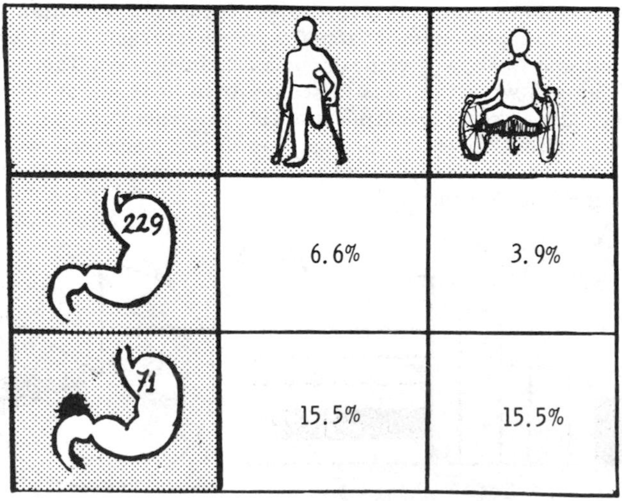

Fig. 40. 'The devil can cite scripture for his purpose' –
The Merchant of Vencie.

Picture charts and combination charts are both useful aids and in commercial advertising they are promoted in journals, where maximal impact must be achieved in a short time. Medical speakers should also employ them for the same effect.

7. Flow Charts

Visual images change continuously just as does our vocabulary. New discoveries bring with them not only new words but new diagrams. The wider use of computers, for instance, popularised the flow chart which has several advantages over conventional diagrams (and may supplement them) for it can –

1. Illustrate successive stages of a process, such as an experiment, from starting point to finish.

2. Be adapted to demonstrate the natural history of a disease. Figure 41 is probably too complex for a single slide and should be made into two.

3. Show a continuous process, such as writing a paper for publication or even planning a lecture and the speaker can take the audience step-by-step down the line.

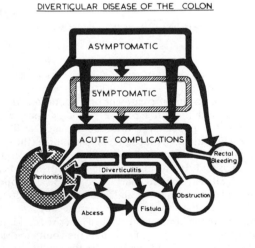

DIVERTICULAR DISEASE OF THE COLON

Fig. 41. 'Stand not upon the order of your going but go at once' – *Macbeth.*

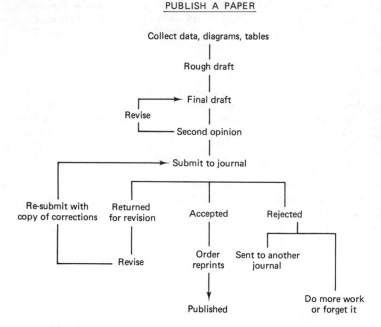

Fig. 42. 'Let there be gall enough in thy ink' – *Twelfth Night*.

4. Aid the art of decision-making in the management of one symptom.

5. Disclose the results of treatment of a condition where patients have been followed up for a precise period of time. Figure 44 is modified from the paper by Clarke, Jones and Needham on the treatment of 433 patients with colorectal carcinoma (the second most common malignant tumour in Britain) from the well-defined area of North-East Scotland. It was published in the British Medical Journal of February 1980. The written chart is too complex for one slide, but the division into two slides (male and female separately) for a lecture is clear cut. We show the flow chart for women only.

6. Demonstrate the family history of an inherited condition quickly and convincingly. The only requirement is the ability to draw straight lines and to use the accepted symbols for the sex of the patients. In many respects this is the original flow chart, although better known under the grand name of 'lineage'.

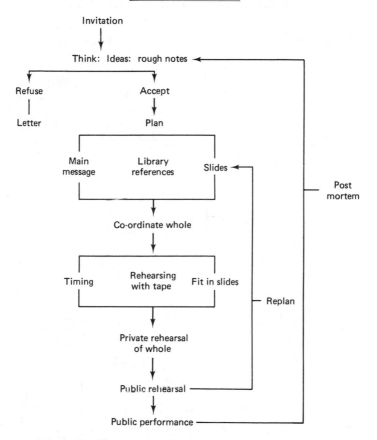

Fig. 43. 'When thy tongue blabs, then let mine eyes not see' –
Twelfth Night.

8. Scatter Graphs

Scatter graphs, or scattergrams, are extremely useful and should be
more widely employed. Many overcrowded column charts (looking
somewhat like the skyline of New York) could easily be turned into
simple scatter graphs. Each single dot represents a value which can be
plotted against one, two, or even three scales (Fig 45)

143

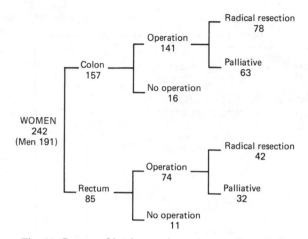

Fig. 44. 'Be sure of it; give me the ocular proof' – *Othello*.

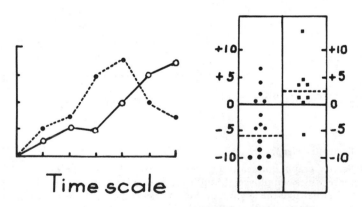

Fig. 45. 'No profit grown where is no pleasure ta'en: in brief, Sir, study what you most affect' – *The Taming of the Shrew*.

The lecturer should be on the look out for new and apt illustrations. He should take the same care in selecting them as he does in choosing the right words. Visual cliches, like worn-out expressions, should be avoided. 'L'image just' delights as much as 'Le mot just'. (For inspiration we recommend the would-be lecturer to look through the books on 'Diagrams' by Lockwood, 'Charts and Graphs' by Simmonds).

9. Photographs

Good clinical photographs enlighten the audience and enliven the lecture. To obtain them you need the combined expertise of a photographer and of a clinician. Ideally, but rarely, these are found in the same person. The next best thing is the physical presence of the clinician at the time of photography, which ensures that the features to be shown are explained to the photographer. His presence also benefits the patient who may find photography embarrassing, uncomfortable and even dangerous.

Photographs of surgical operations may succeed when used to demonstrate a procedure on the surface, such as in plastic, hand or carotid artery surgery. They usually fail when complex procedures are photographed within body cavities, for the camera is not selective enough and cannot 'tidy up the field' for the surgeon. Any audience is usually disorientated when shown a picture through a thoracotomy or laparotomy and the lecture hall seems suddenly filled with a red haze; apart from some gleaming instruments and giant gloved hands, there are no easily recognisable structures on the screen. When we add to this all the difficulties and perhaps the slight dangers (of delay, and of subsequent infection) from photography in the operating room, the use of the camera does not seem worth-while in body cavity surgery. We have seen many ingenious cameras hidden in operating lamps and manipulated by theatre staff, but we have never seen these cameras in use for long. The pictures are disappointing.

Pathological specimens, histological slides and X-rays are highly photogenic and should certainly be used whenever relevant. Indeed, their very attractiveness hides the danger that a lecturer may show a dozen radiological slides when the first two have already conveyed the complete message; or the pathologist may go on providing more pretty pictures of histological preparations than are needed to understand the topic.

10. Diagrams

Diagrams are our favourite form of illustration. A difficult subject can be made easy and the subtle detail of X-ray films highlighted (46A & B). The simpler they are the better. Simplicity of design requires

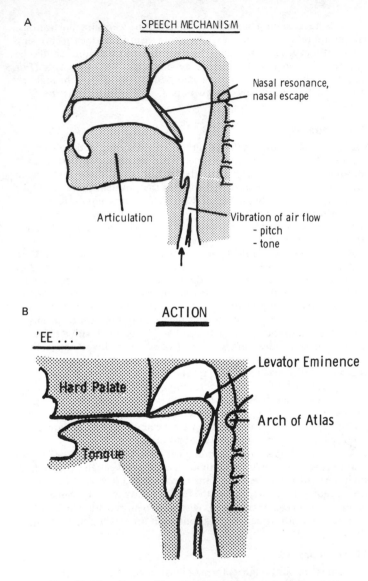

Fig. 46. 'The silence often of pure innocence, persuades when speaking fails' – *The Winter's Tale*.

hard work just as brevity in letter writing requires time; Pascal once wrote, 'I am sorry this letter is so long but I had no time to write a short one'. Similarly, it could be said of a diagram: 'I am sorry this is so complex, but I did not take the trouble to make it simple'. We have already remarked, and would emphasise again, that the labelling of a diagram should be minimal so that it requires the spoken word to explain it.

11. Cartoons

Although we have included humourous drawings in some of our own lectures and in this book, we do not recommend their routine use. Humour is best when it is spontaneous and a drawing prepared in advance and made up as a slide is hardly that. However, a cartoon is not necessarily a sketch trying to be funny; it can also be a simple diagram conveying an idea which may otherwise be difficult to illustrate. For instance, the drawing of a doctor sitting at his desk between two piles of case notes and writing furiously, emphasises that a particular piece of research was retrospective and that it relied on previous records. This cartoon underlines an idea quickly for it is apt and perhaps even witty, without trying to be funny.

12. The Filler Slide

We have mentioned the value of a filler slide earlier, and now give more details about its purpose and design.

There are five reasons for wishing to use filler slides during a lecture:

1. For the shorter lecture we have recommended that the lecturer should show an uninterrupted sequence of slides and not ask for 'lights' half way through. If he does not have enough slides for a continuous flow, the lecturer can put in a blank slide but this will dazzle the audience by so much light from the projector; it is better to mute the brightness by using plain colour.

2. The lecturer who leaves on a slide for too long will lose the attention of the audience while he continues to talk. It is better to change the visual' while continuing with the 'audio'. The filler slide allows just this.

3. When the lecturer wishes to change direction in his talk he may have no slide to indicate this. A filler slide will often quickly alert the audience to the fact that a change is coming and so they will listen more intently.

4. If you wish to summarize what has been said so far, the filler allows projection time for that purpose by providing either no information or a very brief sentence of the conclusions at this stage in the lecture.

5. The filler slide provides time for the lecturer to interject a story, a

reminiscence, a parallel observation, yet keep the full attention of the audience; the idea is to divert their eyes from the screen back to the speaker.

The *design* of the filler slides will depend on the lecture and the occasion. There are at least four different types of slide which any camera enthusiast can make for himself. Some can be used repeatedly in the same lecture or in lectures on different topics. In this sense the filler slide is a general purpose slide; it need not, and perhaps should not, be pointed to. The lecturer must face the audience so that his next few sentences have maximum impact.

1. Plain colours are useful, but they should be pale so that the amount of light around the lecturer is increased and he becomes the focus of attention. A uniform pale grey is recommended by Ollerenshaw but any light colour will do. On the whole blue and red are too vivid and not restful to the eyes.

2. Word summaries – with only a few words on each (we suggest a maximum of seven) – are particularly useful when speaking to an audience largely unknown. When speaking in a foreign country they are mandatory; word summaries may be the only part of the lecture some of the audience will understand. Black lettering on white ground is probably best, again to provide more light around the lecturer while he continues talking.

3. Pictorial views in soft colours make good filler slides. They should contain no distracting objects (such as people, motor cars, houses) so that the scene is taken in quickly by the audience yet remains as a pleasing background to the lecturer. Use mountains, rivers, lakes – those pretty pictures taken on holiday will do nicely.

4. Some filler slides can be used for two purposes: to act as an intermission, and then to indicate new information. For instance, show the photograph of a wall (red brick or Cotswold Stone) and say 'How far have we got? We seem to have reached a brick wall'. Then expand on why, or summarise. The next slide can show the same wall with some key words or a question on it and the lecturer explains how he gets round the impasse. The do-it-yourself enthusiast will photograph a sheet of the appropriate wallpaper and apply bold adhesive lettering – a time-consuming job which will ensure that the number of words is kept to a minimum.

The Use of Colour

Nothing stimulates more argument about slides than colour and Ollerenshaw (1962) concluded that in the choice of colour 'taste and judgement will always be necessary'. Do not try to 'break the monotony' by having different types of slides (white on black, black on

148

white, diazo and colour) as a jumbled lot because they are rarely pleasing together. The audience will guess, correctly, that the slides have been assembled from previous lectures.

Morton (1968) assessed the legibility of various kinds of slides, which he had divided into the following types:

1. Positive – black on white or on a background of colour, such as yellow, green or red.

2. Negative – white on black, or more commonly tinted script on a black background.

3. Diazochrome – white image on a blue or green background.

4. True colour slides.

He found that positive slides (black on white or black on yellow) were more legible than others. We also prefer positive slides but Hawkins (1970) found no preference for positive slides in his experiment with a medical audience.

● The Advantages of Positive Slides

We see the advantages of positive slides as follows:

1. Black on white is familiar and, therefore, not distracting: illustrations in books and students' notes are also black (or dark blue) on white.

2. They are the most legible from a distance. This is our impression which agrees with Morton's scientific findings (and Seymour's conclusions about the light coloured blackboard). Aird (1954) put forward an explanation for this; he suggested that the bright white background forces the eye to adapt by making the pupil contract, so that the smaller aperture for the admission of light increased the depth of focus, as in photography. This may be especially important in the elderly who commonly suffer from some degree of presbyopia.

3. With a white background there is naturally more ambient light and the illumination in the hall need only be dimmed; the lecturer, therefore, does not turn into a disembodied voice in the darkness but remains visible. A further advantage of this semi-darkness is that it allows the audience to take notes easily.

Where the lecture room is large, unknown and the quality of the projector doubtful, black on white slides are the safest to carry: slides, with only 8-12 words on them (and not the 20 allowed) will stand out against the large area of light. If the room cannot be blacked out completely, coloured slides may be illegible even to the lecturer.

4. Finally an ordinary pointer can be used instead of an electric torch to pick out important features on a slide. Colour can, and we believe should be added to positive slides, not for decoration, but to aid understanding. In tables, for instance, the title line should have a coloured background to set it apart from the columns of figures. In a

series of graphs, a recurring curve may be quickly identified if it carries the same colour. Diagrams also benefit from colour, because important details (such as lines of section in an operation, the direction of the flow of fluids circulating in a machine), can be picked out in colour, against the black lines of the rest of the drawing.

- **The Disadvantages of Positive Slides**

1. They are difficult to keep clean. Dust and finger-marks will show on the white or a light coloured background.

2. With positive slides, colours can be achieved only by using colour film. This is expensive. With negative slides, dye can be applied to the slides directly with a fine paint brush.

3. Positive slides take longer to produce while negative, and especially diazochrome transparencies, save considerable time for the photographer.

Lettering

We have already stated that lettering on slides should be kept to a minimum and that in a lecture words are to be spoken and not read.

This is good

THIS IS BETTER AND MORE LEGIBLE.

This is indifferent and uneven

This is easier to read

Fig. 47. 'How use doth breed a habit in a man' –
The Two Gentlemen of Verona.

However, some minimal labelling of most slides is necessary. We repeat the advice that such words on slides must be legible to the naked eye when the slides are held up in the hand; if this is not so, they are likely to be illegible when projected on the screen.

Upper case or capital letters are often used in the mistaken belief that they create emphasis. In practice they are much less legible than lower case letters, a fact which has for long been recognised by the makers of direction signs on motorways and on the Underground. In Fig. 47, lines 1, 2, and 4 were typed on an electric type-writer which provides even pressure and so, better lettering. Lines 2 and 4 were typed on an IBM Executive machine with Director type face: both are infinitely better than line 3 from a manual office machine.

Rules for Slides

To summarise the discussion on individual slides here are 21 points to remember:

1. Do not overcrowd; from one good slide try to make two better ones. If you do have overcrowded slides warn the audience to bring binoculars.

2. Instead of abstract illustrations, verbal slides and tables, try to think up diagrams and cartoons.

3. Make them simple and pictorial. Emphasize one point only; hence you may have to distribute the total information over several slides. If this means six slides are you trying to do too much in the time available?

4. Avoid verbal slides; in a talk, words are to be heard not to be seen and read. If you must use them, limit the number to 20 words or less.

5. Labelling should be minimal and lettering in lower case.

6. Avoid tables. If you must use them observe the 3 rules.

7. Graphs or curve charts are used to express changes against time: plot only one, or at the most two, curves on a single graph.

8. Column, bar and pie charts are for making comparisons; select the most appropriate for your data.

9. Use special statistical slides only when appropriate and then always explain them fully.

10. Remember, when using photographs, that not all subjects are equally photogenic.

11. Do not waste space on the transparencies: fill the whole viewing area.

12. Use colour with purpose and not for mere decoration.

13. Use bold dry transfer figures on X-ray films and always cut out any excess film before making the slide. This will also magnify the area you really want to show.

14. Never use serial numbers on slides. The audience will wonder why number 20 comes before number 11. Avoid dates if possible.

15. Never be in the position when you have to say, cheerfully or sadly: 'Disregard the top two-thirds of this slide. Just concentrate on the bottom part'. You have failed yourself and your audience. Courtesy and consideration demand a slide for the occasion, not a left-over from some previous event.

16. If you need to refer to a slide shown earlier never ask the projectionist to back-track. Always have a duplicate to insert at the right place.

17. Each letter should be 5% of the height of the artwork for good visibility.

18. Above all, decide what you want to show (a general idea or specific detail) and how you want to show it. If you are not clear in your own mind, no slide will do the job of thinking for you.

19. If a slide is shown back-to-front (your fault and not the projectionist's) then you can either ask for it to be put right, which may require more than one attempt (there are at least four ways of getting it wrong), or you can accept the inconvenience and shrug it off: why not say 'this slide is labelled in Russian, but I will point out the important features', or, 'we decided to photograph the patient upside-down to make it easier for you to see that . . .'? Such impromptu remarks add flavour to a lecture and show that the speaker is in control: we don't recommend them, but realise that we live in an imperfect world.

20. Omit all unnecessary detail – at the planning and production stage, not during the lecture. Make your slides attractive and eye-catching. Note how the Ad. man does it.

21. If a slide tells the complete story, keep quiet; do not read out, do not point, but allow time for the audience to absorb the information, to make an assessment, to place the information in the correct and logical order of the lecture, to appreciate what it means, and to work out what is likely to follow. All this requires 20 to 40 seconds, even for a good slide. The wise lecturer will use the pause to think of what he will say next.

9

VISUAL AIDS III
DO-IT-YOURSELF

'There are four things that make this world go round: love, energy, materials, and information. We see about us a critical shortage of the first commodity, a near critical shortage of the second, increasing shortage of the third, but an absolute glut of the fourth.'
Robert A. Day (1979)

From the Royal Postgraduate Medical School and Hammersmith Hospital come about 600 publications every year: scientific advances, reviews, case reports. If, on average, each paper requires about four charts (tables, diagrams, graphs) the total is staggering: we would need three full-time illustrators to cope with that load alone. In addition there are about four times the number of lectures given, where the demand for visual information is greater. Because of these large numbers, Doig Simmonds set up a do-it-yourself studio in 1976 so that lecturers could seek expert advice and then produce their own artwork: the resulting products have been excellent and the amateurs have enjoyed learning a great deal. There are plenty of books to help the D.I.Y. householder, but few for the lecturer and writer in medicine (consult Price, 1969: Simmonds, 1980; Reynolds and Simmonds, 1981) to fill this deficiency.

There are three things the amateur can do just as well as the professional, with a little practice and a lot of patience: drawings, clinical photographs and slides, all of which can be made cheaply and quickly by anyone who has not the services of a medical artist.

Making your own Drawings

The first step in drawing diagrams is to obtain the right tools. These are:

1. Pencil and rubber,
2. Ruler and ruling pen,
3. Coloured felt tip pens with fine tips,
4. India ink, which is black and waterproof,
5. A No. 1 water colour sable brush and a tube of poster white.
6. Smooth illustration board (this is superior to paper and stands up to rough handling),
7. Transfer sheets with alphabets, symbols and shading (e.g. Letraset and Letratone).

8. Toilet paper, soft tissue. One snap and you have the right sized piece to wipe pens clean: a jam jar of water will keep them fresh.

A drawing should start with a pencil sketch. A great deal of trail and error, rubbing out and re-drawing is to be expected at this stage. Once the final pencil sketch is arrived at it should be inked over and, when the India ink has dried, the pencil lines are rubbed out.

Ink lines should be drawn evenly and without jerks. The whole arm, and especially the hand, must be well supported on the table. The pen is moved deliberately, neither too fast nor too slow. A curved outline is best drawn in sections, leaving tiny gaps between adjacent strokes. For each section the position of the resting arm should be moved so that the movement of fingers and wrist is least constricted and most natural while following the curve of a particular line. Care should be taken not to smudge the still wet ink, but blots or mistakes can easily be covered with poster white. Errors in the construction of graphs are almost inevitable; these too can be deleted with the brush and white paint. Dotted lines are best obtained by drawing a continuous line and breaking it up with poster white. This saves time and gives a squared off finish at the beginning and end of each dash or dot.

Lettering used to be the artist's nightmare but the introduction of transfer alphabets, and the electric typewriter, have brought this within the capacity of even the amateur. Not only letters in various sizes and types, but numbers and symbols, such as arrows, circles and squares are now available on transfer sheets such as Letraset and Letratone.

Shading is frequently required in graphs and diagrams. This too can be obtained in an endless variety of transfer sheets but make shading bold. They are easily employed by removing the backing sheet, applying the shading over the area to be filled and then burnishing it on the diagram, preferably with an empty ball-point pen. A scalpel is used to cut the transfer along the edges of the shaded area and the excess is gently peeled off.

Any 35mm camera may be used to photograph the completed drawing. Colour transparency film, having little grain, is satisfactory both for black and white, and for coloured originals. A further advantage is that the colour film can be sent off to the developers and is returned made up into mounted transparencies, and therefore ready for showing.

● The Special Value of Drawings

Simple line drawings have eight useful qualities. They are easy to execute and can provide:

1. Illustration of things that photography cannot. For instance,

many skin conditions are highly photogenic. But deep inside the abdomen, photography often shows large hands retracting tissues, much gore, and a poorly identified stricture of the large bowel. Drawings do the job better and have more impact. In this respect we acknowledge Leonardo da Vinci as the first medical illustrator: unfortunately few imitate him.

2. Information about the real world: not just about strictures deep in the abdomen, but to demonstrate features which on an X-ray film would be difficult to see.

3. Abstract ideas. Here we come back to the principle of instant recognition. If you are talking about cancer of the breast and wish to show the results of treatment (mean and standard deviations of course) then a simple diagram will alert the audience to the stage of the disease and hold their attention, while you discuss the specific detail that you are trying to put across. The motif can be repeated on a series of slides.

4. Something for the audience to copy into a notebook quickly. It is almost impossible to sketch from a photograph within the time available.

5. An impression of movement by adding dotted lines (of full function) to the bolder outline of the static condition.

6. The impact of maps (of distribution of populations and their diseases) which no other method does quite as well. Tables are boring compared with a simple line diagram and appropriate shading.

7. Diagrams can provide a message very quickly and hence allow the lecturer to use several to put over his message. Recently, we attended a 10-minute lecture on the variations of the Roux-en-Y duodenal loop and their uses. This is a rather technical subject even for an audience of general surgeons. The lecturer wisely provided 15 unlabelled diagrams. He realised that the liver, the gallbladder, the stomach and the duodenum all have distinctive shapes, instantly recognisable. He, therefore, explained the surgical procedure during the showing of the first diagram and then whizzed through the rest with minimal comment. To have tried to put all this on word slides would have been fatal; to have labelled each one would have diverted the interest of the audience. Moreover, everyone listening understood the message: the Roux-en-Y loop is a very versatile procedure (the message came across!).

8. Simple line drawings can be used as background to pathological specimens to orientate the viewer. India ink outlines, thicker than usual size, on A4 glazed white cards, can be drawn of the skull, jaw, neck, pelvis, abdomen. The specimen removed at operation is then dried and laid on the drawing. The whole can be photographed in colour or black-and-white, to make attractive and informative slides. The technique requires imagination, little skill, but a flair for lighting

so that shadows are correctly placed to give a three-dimensional effect. No labelling is required.

● Rules for drawings

1. Reduce the content to bare essentials. The cartoonist draws lines and then rubs out those which the imagination of the viewer will fill in mentally. Imitate him. A schematic form is pleasing.

2. Do not include any detail which you do not intend to comment on.

3. Divide the complicated into simple portions, which usually means more than one slide. Give an overall picture by all means, but do not comment on this: ask for the 'next slide' immediately and then describe the detail.

4. Simplify every diagram.

5. Use thick lines (at least 0.5mm) for contrast, use no minute details and no half tones. Use large symbols (dots, circles, crosses) and use different symbols for each value, but be consistent throughout.

6. Be bold.

7. Try to work within a small format, say 6 × 9cm, because this will make you lay out your drawings in the most simple way. If you use the same format, all slides will appear to be uniform in composition.

8. Provide instant recognition.

9. Convert tables to graphs, to histograms, to bar-charts or to pie-diagrams to see which provides the greatest impact. In other words, play the 'conversion game'.

10. Use minimal lettering. Do not spell out words when you intend to describe them: simplify by single letters.

11. Aim to have a maximum of seven lines on a slide with not more than 25 characters on each line (which includes spacing). Even this is too much for most lectures. Choose the style of lettering with care. The rub-on letters, so easy to use, are not very artistic. Where possible use type-face of Gothic or Univers, which we prefer.

12. Choose the background with purpose. Black lettering on white background dazzles, but allows the lecturer to be in full view of the audience throughout the lecture. Coloured backgrounds (blue, red, green) dazzle and tire the eyes much less, but colour can be monotonous. The present fashion for diazo slides will fade, thankfully: the lettering is often sub-standard and the colour tone not the same on every slide (partly the effect of ageing, partly from exposure to light, partly from faults in the development process).

290 cm	
111 cm	Use Stencils No typing

21 cm	
14 cm	General format Type or stencil

12 cm	
8 cm	Tables

9 cm	
6 cm	Word slides

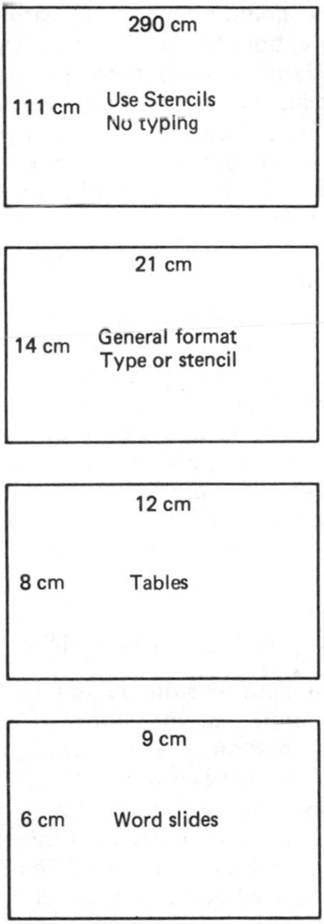

Fig. 48. 'Suit the action to the word, the word to the action, with special observance, that you o'erstep not the modesty of nature' – *Hamlet.*

Taking your own Clinical Photographs

Always carry a camera. There are many situations where a colour shot could be taken so easily and used later as a slide to highlight the content of a lecture. Such occasions tend not to be repeated, so it is safer to have a camera at hand. Cameras are bulky. Since a flash is also

157

necessary, some form of case to hold the equipment, extra film and a notebook to record details of each exposure, become essential.

The 35mm camera should be of quality with a good lens – f2.8 is sufficient for most situations but an f1.5 has advantages; through-the-lens viewing is mandatory for amateurs and one with a light meter incorporated has great advantages. The investment in an expensive camera pays handsome dividends, once the owner really knows how to use it and knows his limitations. There are several excellent and cheap manuals of instruction marketed by the film manufacturers which will help the novice to get started.

● **Rules for photographs**

1. Make sure that important features stand out. So, a broad general view followed by a close-up is frequently required. The broad view orientates the viewer, the close-up provides the essential detail.

2. The background should contain no distractions, such as a clock, light switches, posters, doors, other people and other equipment. This often means that the amateur photographer has to provide his own background: a cloth sheet (we prefer pale blue, but pale green will do) or a roll of plain paper will suffice, but remember that colour may be important – white skin on a dark background looks well, but black skin will not.

Making your own slides

You may think that because you do not have the facilities of a professional photographic unit you cannot produce good slides. Not so. You will need a tripod and camera, some knowledge, and much patience. The camera should be chosen with care. For copying artwork you may need a lens which will photograph crisply at about nine inches: most 50mm lens only do the job at three feet. But there is range called 'macro' lenses of 50/55mm or 100/105mm which will do the job well, usually providing a half reduction, sometimes a one-to-one ratio. A single lens reflex (SLR) is essential and an in-built exposure meter useful. One way round the problem is to buy additional lenses to attach but on the whole extension rings are better because the need for extra glass (and its problems) are avoided. The financial outlay will be repaid quickly and pleasurably by first class productions. There are three methods for the amateur:

1. Ordinary black and white film to produce negatives (white lettering on a black background which is rarely completely opaque). Panchromatic film of fine grain, say FP4, can be bought from any photographic shop. The white lettering can be tinted although it is difficult to produce an even colour: the tint may show through the

background (because that is not densely black). Colour is added using spirit-based felt-tipped pens – red, green, blue – as used for writing on acetate film for the overhead projector; Stabilo or Edding 1200 both write well on glass. It is not easy to obtain uniform colouring. You may find water-based pens easier to use because you can 'build up' colour by wiping over again and again: they take well on film emulsion, and do not dry quickly on the pen. Use the Staedtler range (Marsmatic 700), available from graphic artist suppliers. Films can also be dipped in solutions, and yellow is the best, but they are expensive: it is also difficult to prevent a streaky effect which looks amateurish. Alternatively the negative film (or positive) can be mounted together with pale coloured gel sheets as used for stage lighting.

2. Direct reversal film, to give black letters on a white background: Agfa-Gevaert Dia Direct film is processed by the manufacturer; Kodak SO 185 is processed by an agency, or it can be developed in the X-omat tank of the hospital X-ray department. Both are available from professional photographic shops; again slow speeds, useful for reproduction of X-rays (illuminated from a light box, with black paper masking of non-essentials) because the contrasts are the same as on the originals whereas ordinary black-and-white film will reverse them.

3. Colour slide positive film, such as Kodachrome, Ektachrome or Agfachrome: for the last two there are processing kits for the keen amateur, otherwise all are processed by the manufacturer or agencies. The film speeds are variable. Kodachrome has a finer grain than Ektachrome, but you can photograph X-rays (a greenish tinge) and black and white art-work; for the latter you can use various colour filters – yellow, blue, red – to give black letters on a different ground, but the filters will alter the exposure time.

Not only is the making of one's own slides cheaper, it is often quicker and more satisfying. The cost per frame from standard 36 exposure film works out at about fourpence for panchromatic, fivepence for reversal and twelvepence for colour: a ratio of three-to-one against colour which may be the most useful because the end of the roll can be used to make filler slides; either you can photograph a series of different coloured sheets of paper (wallpaper will do) or one white sheet using various filters. Better still take some local scenes. For the beginner, it is advisable to take several shots at different apertures to be sure of one good picture; the small extra expense is worthwhile, for a really good slide goes a long way to making a successful lecture.

Finally, a note about lighting. Lighting of the object must be even. Using a flash is too difficult for the amateur. It is better to use natural lighting – bright overcast or if a sunny day then go into shadow to work. Alternatively, use four photoflood lamps on a stand over the object, but this becomes semi-professional and produces problems of its own.

Some manufacturers produce a quite extensive range of systems for copying; they are expensive (cheapest £600) and a poor investment for the occasional photographer.

In photographing your own artwork for slides we recommend O'Neill's nine technical points:

1. Keep the film plane parallel with the orignal, by using a spirit level on the back of the camera.

2. Make sure that what you are copying lies flat.

3. Check that the lighting is even, with no bright spots, dim areas or flare (light going directly on to the lens).

4. If using colour film make sure that the quality of lighting is correct: if not then use filters to match.

5. Use a lens which will produce a sharp image for close-ups, because most copying will be of that sort.

6. Beware of reflections from shiny materials either from the artwork paper or from the sheet of glass used to keep it flat.

7. Use a polarising filter on the lens for maximum contrast when using colour.

8. Watch out for subtle problems which may spoil the results: ageing bulbs, drop in voltage, long exposures.

9. Put in some practice and experiments before planning to produce all your own slides.

Slide check – before making them

There is one invariable rule: check everything before you photograph it. Professional carpenters are told to 'measure twice, cut once'. The DIY handyman learns the hard way, but the advice certainly applies to lecturers. Double check the artwork before filming. And by artwork we mean every illustration – tables, graphs, histograms, word slides, diagrams, cartoons, drawings (particularly your own) – the lot.

The commonest fault with a slide projected on the day of the lecture is to find an error of spelling or calculation. If a word is spelt incorrectly and the lecturer recognises it for the first time, this will halt his flow of speech. He will often apologise to the audience who will have spotted it immediately. Our advice is don't: ignore it. If you can't ignore it, then do not apologise; it is better to say that you have never been able to spell the word 'legible' correctly and that your secretary, who typed it, has such faith in you that she refused to alter a single word.

If numerical data are incorrect on the slide, that is a more serious matter. To have to explain to the audience that '0.2 should be 7.5', to take an extreme example (but such gross errors happen still) is a cardinal sin. The audience will begin to doubt the veracity of all that you say, as indeed they should. If you have followed our rules and advice then the following 20 questions will help in selecting the lecture slides:

1. Does the slide give essential information?
2. Is the visual information likely to be understandable to others?
3. Is the information immediately recognisable?
4. Has the content been trimmed to the bare essentials?
5. Are there any distractions still apparent?
6. Does the written commentary conflict with information on the slide?
7. Will the slide appeal to the intended audience?
8. Has it been simplified enough?
9. Have important features been emphasised?
10. Are there clear enough contrasts between colours/light and dark?
11. Is the lettering clearly legible?
12. Will abstract signs be recognisable, or are they unusual and require explanation?

INSTANT RECOGNITION

Cancer of the breast

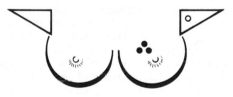

Treatment (& No. patients)	Mean survival In months (+ S.D.)
A (100)	C (+ e)
B (100)	D (+ f)
A v B	P =

Fig. 49. 'Find out the course of this effect, or rather say, the cause of this defect, for this effect defective comes by cause' – *Hamlet*.

13. Are abbreviations obvious?

14. Are numerical tables necessary or could they be converted to diagrams?

15. Will the slide communicate important knowledge to that particular audience?

16. Has the whole slide area been used effectively?

17. Would an extra slide help to get the message over?

18. What slide could be omitted?

19. Are words correctly spelt, is everything in order?

20. Murphy's Law applies to slides: if something can go wrong, it will. We have recommended that the lecturer should arrive early for his lecture, should look through his slides before handing them to the projectionist, should spend a few minutes in quiet contemplation before making his appearance. We now suggest that he should ask himself another question: what could go wrong and how will he recover?

Our check list may seem dogmatic, it is. But the final criterion is this: if you can read your own slide at arms length then it will be clear to all members of the audience when projected. What is on the slide is your affair, and for judgement by others.

Using the Medical Artist

Life is too short to do everything oneself; we cannot all become like Leonardo da Vinci, scientist and artist, Jack of all trades. If you have an illustration department use it and use it well. A bit of do-it-yourself in the past may help you here, for you will then appreciate the difficulties of the professional. There are two things to remember in asking for his co-operation:

1. Take the artist fully into your confidence; explain what you want to illustrate and why. Make sketches of your plans but invite and accept his criticism. When asking for clinical photographs do not rely alone on written instructions to the photographer; it is better to go and see him in person and, if at all possible, to be present at the actual photography.

2. Give him plenty of warning: if you have tried it yourself, you will know just how time-consuming it all is. Most departments have a heavy work load, with bursts of extra activities just before a meeting or symposium. It is therefore good advice to have your illustrations prepared before all the other speakers start competing for the same artist and the same photographer.

Storing and Transporting Slides

The itinerant and regular speaker will soon acquire a number of slides for various lectures. He will also have collected slides of patients, experiments, people and places of interest for possible future use. What is he to do with them? All should be labelled, filed in a convenient place and kept away from direct sunlight.

It is usually better to number the slides in sequence as they accumulate and to use a card index or book for their retrieval. There are four methods of storage:

1. In boxes, labelled sequentially so that the individual boxes fit into a cabinet. Surgical sutures are dispatched in polystyrene boxes with a sliding lid and these hold about 45 slides. Since the boxes are disposable, every hospital operating theatre has a supply which would otherwise be thrown away. This is the cheapest and simplest method of storage but it does not allow easy selection of an appropriate slide by inspection.

2. 'Slidepak' transparency filing wallets have a 41cm long bar at the top and can be hung in a standard filing cabinet. They are made of clear P.V.C. and hold 24, 5 × 5cm mounted slides. When lifted up to the light the content can easily be seen, but a magnifying glass is an asset for detailed viewing. The filing wallets can also be laid flat on a lighted X-ray viewing box so that arrangement of the sequence of slides for a lecture becomes a simple matter. The metal bar can be removed and the whole folded to fit into the coat pocket for transportation; it is advisable, however, to place them in a dustproof envelope before doing so.

3. The 'Fogro' wallets are also made of clear P.V.C. and will hold 50 mounted 5 × 5 slides, to fold into an area 29 × 6 × 3cm. They are thus more convenient for transportation, but rather expensive for storage unless it is desired to store the requirements of an individual lecture separately.

4. Larger boxes of wood or cardboard in which each slide has its special slot. These are made to take 100 to 200 slides.

Slides should never be carried loose in the pocket. They will only collect dust, the glass covers may become broken and the important labelling, serial number and identification spot will wear thin. They should be carried either in one of the storage devices or in a separate, suitable, firm and dust-free container. If only a few slides are required then either pack the empty space of the box with clean paper to ensure that the slides do not fall out of the correct order, or use a smaller container such as that returned with developed colour films.

Final Preparations Before a Lecture

A speaker arriving just before the start of his talk is unlikely to give a really good lecture. Commonly, after passing his slides to the projectionist at the last minute, he will trip over the pointer, drop his notes on the podium, search for light switches and then accidentally press the wrong ones, cause blinds to shut, electric fans to hum into life and large epidiascopes to rise out of the ground. His mistakes may be less amusing; when asking for the first slide, the one with the final conclusions will appear on the screen, the rest will be out of order, some even upside-down, and all will be dirty and thumbmarked. Some of his slides may seem to surprise him, and after a few seconds of stunned silence he will mumble, 'Oh, yes . . . well, I think we can skip this one today'.

To avoid such a shambles we recommend a few minutes quiet meditation with one's slides preferably on the morning of the lecture; they should be cleaned with an anti-static cloth (obtainable from your local chemist, optician or photographic dealer). They should be cleaned carefully and put in order, numbered and labelled afresh for this particular occasion.

Adhesive paper labels should be stuck on the right-hand upper corner of the mount next to the permanent marker on the slides, and they should be listed numerically on a card with a short description of

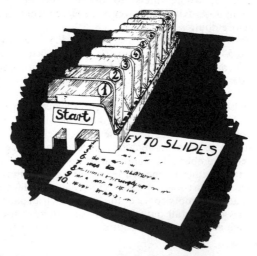

Fig. 50. 'This is the very coinage of your brain' – *Hamlet*.

each. This card will remain with the speaker, so that if need be, he can ask for a slide by number, while on the podium.

The slides must be handed over to the projectionist well in advance, in a container bearing the name of the speaker and the title of the lecture. The container should also be marked to indicate the 'start' of the sequence. Now the speaker can settle down and reconnoitre his locale. When his turn comes he will know how to present his slides to their best advantage.

10
THE 10 COMMANDMENTS

'By their fruits ye shall know them.'
Matthew 7.20

1. Look good and feel good. Be alive and alert, but never be arrogant.
2. Speak clearly and don't read.
3. Prepare thoroughly. Disguise the fact that you have spent more time in preparation than the audience deserves.
4. Allow sufficient time.
5. Rehearse frequently.
6. Arrange sequences logically, use language correctly.
7. Be selective in material.
8. Use the appropriate visual aid.
9. Entertain, inform, educate – in that order, but include all three.
10. Be friendly, humorous and kindly. Give the impression that you are enjoying the occasion. Answer questions with charity.

11

FURTHER READING, REFERENCES, MATERIALS

*'Some books are to be tasted, others to be swallowed, and some few
to be chewed and digested . . . Reading maketh an exact man.'*
Francis Bacon

The best way to be in a position to judge issues is to read around them.
There are three basic types of reading:

1. General textbooks on the art of public speaking. There are many
on the market and probably some in your local public library. Consult
the librarian.

2. Specialised reading which may go into greater depth than you
need. It is often necessary to confine reading to a few chapters; for
instance, in books on speech training, voice production, drama,
business studies, and so on. Just read those pieces which bear on the
subject of public speaking. So browse among the library shelves.

3. Journals often contain articles on lecturing, organisation of
symposia and related subjects. Look for such papers in the British
Medical Journal, Lancet, Science, Journal of Medical Education,
New England Journal of Medicine, Journal of the American Medical
Association, and several others. Photocopy or make notes from the
most helpful papers, for use later.

The only way to judge a lecture is to go and listen, but knowledge of
technique will help. In the end, if you wish to speak well you have to
make the effort, not just think about it.

References and Reading

Aird I., Quoted by Ollerenshaw R., (1962)
Bacharach A.L., Communications at meetings in general. *The Analyst*
1954; **79**: 530-4. (Excellent summary of vices and virtues in lecturing
particularly for the short scientific communication).
Barabas A., Blackboard Drawing in Medical Teaching. *Brit med J*
1965; **1**: 782-4.
Barabas A., On lecturing. *Brit J Hosp Med* 1974 (**Sept**); 320-2.
Brinkman G., Diazo slides. *Med Biol Illus* 1964; **14**: 299-301.
Brook B.N., Audio-visual aids in the medical school. *Lancet* 1970; **2**:
817. (Dogma disputed: Argues against the excessive reliance on films
and television.)

Beard R.M., *Research into teaching methods in higher education.* 1968. Research into Higher Education Ltd., 2 Woburn Square, London, WC1. (Useful chapters on 'the lecture', on 'audio-visual aids', and on 'selection and evaluation of teaching methods', includes comprehensive list of references).

Calnan J., A lecture on lecturing. *Medical Education* 1976; **10**: 445-9.

C.I.O.M.S. Union of International Meetings 1967. (Discusses all aspects of organising large medical congresses and conferences: deals briefly with small symposia: interesting observations on the psychology of 'participants behaviour'.)

De Bakey L., *The scientific journal. Editorial policies and practices. Guidelines for editors, reviewers and authors.* C.V. Mosby: St. Louis, 1976.

Evans M., The abuse of slides. *Brit Med J* 1978; **2**: 905-8.

Eyre E.C., *Effective communication made simple.* Allen: London, 1979. (Deals with all forms of communication, but useful chapters on speaking.)

Flint M.F., *A user's guide to copyright.* Butterworths: London 1979.

Grann V., Interest patient syndrome. *Arch Int Med* 1965; **116**: 442-3.

Gunning R., *The technique of clear writing.*
McGraw-Hill; New York, 1968. (Read his 'Fog Index').

Hansell P., and Ollerenshaw R., *Longmore's medical photography* 8th Ed. The Focal Press: London, 1978. (A classic work for the medical photographer).

Hawkins C.F., *Speaking and writing in medicine.*
Thomas: Philadelphia; 1967.

Kodak publications. Effective Lecture Slides, No. S-22. *Planning, preparation, and legibility in the production of transparencies for projection.* No. AV-6.

Kraft A.R., Saletta J.D., Moss G.S., Herman C.M., and Tomkins R.K., A critical appraisal of the effectiveness of scientific presentations. *J Surg Res* 1976; **20**: 377-9. (Makes depressing reading, but must be read.)

Lawrence R.S., *A guide to speaking in public.* Pan Books: London, 1979. (Full of good sense.)

Leech R, *Give a lecture in HOW TO DO IT.* British Medical Association: London, 1979.

Littleton L.T., Cartooning in medical illustration. *J. Guthrie Clin Bull* 1969; **39**: 14-18.

Lockwood A., *Diagrams.* Studio-Vista: London, 1967. (A visual encyclopaedia of diagrams with 250 illustrations in 144 pages).

Manten A.A., *Symposia and symposium publication: a guide for organisers, lecturers and editors of scientific meetings.* Elsevier: Amsterdam, 1976.

Meadow R., Speaking at medical meetings. *Lancet* 1969; **2**: 631-3. (Excellent article; recommended reading.)

Meyer-Hartwig K., Bleifeld W., and Hegewald U., *How to compose slides for lectures.* Witzstrock: Baden-Baden 1977. (An illustrated guide, easy to follow.)

Minor E., and Frye H.R., *Techniques for producing visual instructional media.* McGraw-Hill: London, 1970.

Mitchell J., *How to write reports.* Fontana: Glasgow, 1974.

Morton R., The lantern slide. *Photographic J* 1969; **108**: 89-92.

Ollerenshaw R., Design for projection: a study of legibility. *Photographic J* 1962; **101**: 147-54.

Ollerenshaw R., and Hansell P., Some medical aids to instruction. *Brit Med J* 1950; **2**: 488-93.

O'Neill J.P., 101 ways to make copy and title slides . . . some of them good. *J Biol Photog Assoc.* 1978; **41**: 141-52.

Price F., Medical illustration on a do-it-yourself basis. *Proc Roy Soc Med* 1969; **62**: 815-7.

Rathbone R.R., *Communicating technical information* 3rd Ed. Addison-Wesley: Reading, Mass, 1972. (Originally published in 1966, now in its third printing with revisions. A short book full of sound advice.)

Reynolds L., and Simmonds D., *Presentation of data in science: principles and practices for authors and teachers.* Nijhoff: The Hague, 1981.

Shephard D.A.E., How to evaluate papers given at medical meetings: use of the SPEAKER Index. *Brit Med J* 1979; **4**: 1403-4. (An original idea for the assessment of an everyday occurrence).

Seymour W.D., An experiment showing the superiority of a light coloured blackboard. *Brit J Educational Psychology*, 1937; **7**: 259-61.

Simmonds D., Ed. *Charts and graphs: guidelines for the visual presentation of statistical data in the life sciences.* Published in association with the Institute of Medical and Biological Illustrations. MTP Press: Lancaster, 1980.

Taggart P., Carruthers M., and Sommerville W., Electrocardiograms, plasma catecholamines and lipids, and their modification by oxyprenolol when speaking before an audience. *Lancet* 1973; **2**: 341-6. (Must be read, even by the nervous.)

Vincent A., *The overhead projector.* Report No. 8. The Experimental Development Unit of the National Committee for Audio-Visual Aids in Education, 33 Queen Anne Street, London W1M 0AL. (Examines all aspects of the overhead projector and recommend it for small group teaching. Titles of other monographs can be noted from the same series and may be obtained from the above address. The same committee also published digests of articles on audio-visual aids under the title 'Survey of British Research in Audio-Visual Aids').

Warren P.J., New concepts in lecture theatre control systems for medical schools. *Brit J med Educn* 1972; **6**: 301-5.

Whitwam J.G., Spoken communication. *Brit J Anaesth* 1970; **42**: 768-78.

Williams P.C., *Suggestions for speakers and standards for slides.* Reprinted from Institute of Biology Journal. May 1965.

Wright A., *Designing for visual aids.* Studio Vista: London, 1970. (In just under 100 pages deals with visual aids in education; the theory of learning; the various types of visual aids from slides to television, and the designing of visual aids in general.)

Zollinger R.M. and Howe C.T., The illustration of medical lectures. *Med Biol Illus* 1964; **14**: 154-7.

Essential Reference Books

The first three books are well worth buying, or at least having readily available:

1. A good dictionary. *Chambers* or the *Shorter Oxford* dictionary (in two volumes, easier to manage) for the meaning of words. What you utter may not mean what you say: so check with the dictionary. A good exercise is to open a dictionary at random and read the definitions of simple words: some definitions are antiquated, others passing, some modern, others ahead of current usage. Consult medical dictionaries such as *Dorlands* (Saunders, Philadelphia) and *Butterworths* (MacNalty A.S. ed.) for medical words.

2. *Roget's Thesaurus of English Words and Phrases* (Penguin Books, London), for alternative and more forceful words. This is a book of synonyms, but in English a synonym may not convey the exact connotation you wish. The value of the Thesaurus lies (we believe) mainly in stimulating thought: often the right word comes quite suddenly after perusing the pages and may not be included. So, a book for getting the context going rather than a simple word-exchanger.

3. *Fowler's Modern English Usage*: to be dipped into, to find constructions, examples and errors in the use of language. If a word 'sticks' in the script as being awkward then look it up in Fowler.

4. A good book of quotations (such as Bartlett), the complete Shakespeare and The Bible.

5. For humour, read the short stories of James Thurber (*The Thurber Carnival* in three volumes); Missen L., *Quotable Anecdotes*: Allen; London 1966; and Prochnow H.V., and Prochnow H.V. Jr. *The Public Speakers Treasure Chest.* Thomas: Preston, 1965.

6. Access, by your local library, to *Encyclopaedia Britannica, Chambers Encyclopedia, Pears* annual encyclopaedia, *Whittakers* annual Almanac (all for details of world events, dates and tit-bits of unexpected information).

7. For medical men of stature, read Strauss M.R., *Familiar Medical Quotations*. Little, Brown & Co: Boston, 1968 and Morton L.T., *Medical Bibliography*. 3rd Edn Deutsch: London, 1970.

8. A box file of your own references – cuttings from newspapers, magazines, journals, notes on the back of envelopes – which are difficult to file in any sort of order: so just throw them in one box and, before a lecture, browse through the lot.

9. Finally, a little black pocket book in which to record quotations heard on the radio, television, other people's lectures, after-dinner speeches, in the wards, as well as apt phrases read in journals, newspapers and books. The same small pocket book (which should be examined thoroughly once a month) can also have jottings for possible lectures in the future: subjects, observations and hypotheses should all be included – one item to each page will allow space for those brilliant ideas which come later.

Materials

1. Fogro folding wallets for 35mm slides are obtainable from most photographic retailers. An A4 size 'book' to hold 600 slides of various lectures is available from Koroseal Trading Co., 225 Southwark Bridge Road, London SE1 0DN.

2. 'Viewpack' storage folders of clear polythene with pockets to hold 12, 20 or 24 slides supplied by Diana Wyllie Ltd., 3 Park Road, Baker Street, London NW1 and 'Slidepack' folders for hanging in standard filing cabinets supplied by Roneo Vickers Ltd.

3. Epidiascope white cards: A.G. Bishop, Stationary Supplies, St. Mary Cray, Orpington, Kent.

4. Pocket tape-recorders are relatively cheap and most useful for private rehearsal of lectures. The quality of sound matters little but the ease of playback does: Philips 85 'Pocket Memo', or Grundig EN3L 'Electronic notebook'. Both companies have world-wide distribution, and both use the simple but different cassette tapes. It is advantageous to choose the same make as that of other recording equipment in your office or institution.

5. Fluorescent chalks from The American Crayon Company, Sandusky, Ohio, New York State, under the name of Prang Excello Squares.

6. Fluorescent lighting: Theatre Project Services Limited, 10-16 Mercer Street, London WC2 – order lamp No. 230C, with tripod stand.

7. Acetate film and holders, from Gordon Audio Visual Limited, 28-30 Market Place, Oxford Circus, London W1N 8PH.

12

APPENDIX

We include, as an appendix, the printed sheets sent as guidelines to all those who submit and give papers to the Surgical Research Society. They are produced here by kind permission of a Society which regularly maintains a high standard of presentation at meetings and has acted to preserve it.

We commend them to others who may have to arrange their own meetings, symposia, conferences and work-shops in the future with the hope that organisers will take note and enforce better discipline on their own speakers.

SURGICAL RESEARCH SOCIETY

PREPARATION OF SUMMARIES – REVISED INSTRUCTIONS

IMPORTANT: THIS INSTRUCTION SHEET MUST BE STRICTLY ADHERED TO, and members submitting summaries are requested to ensure that they conform to the following requirements.

1. TEN (10) COPIES of each summary should be submitted
    - the text must not exceed 200 words
    - typed on ONE A4 SHEET IN DOUBLE SPACING

2. The Title of the paper should precede the text on every copy.

3. ON THREE (3) COPIES ONLY:
    - author(s) initials and surname(s) in that order should be given but no titles or degrees
    - in joint authorship, the name of the person who will read the paper must be placed first
    - if none of the authors is a member of the Society, the name of the member introducing the paper must be added, in brackets, after the name(s) of the author(s)
    - the Department, Institute and Place (e.g. London) should be stated. Postal codes will not be included in the published summaries.

4. Indicate at the top right hand corner of all ten (10) copies whether the abstract is being submitted either for "presentation" or for the "poster" session.

5. Indication of grant support will not be published in abstracts and should not be included.

6. **IMPORTANT FOOTNOTE.** At the end of the *top* copy of each summary the following note should be added:

    a) The work described in this summary has/has not been previously published. (If already published, please give name of Journal).

    b) The work contained in this summary has/has not been read at a scientific meeting. (If so, please give details).

    c) The work described in this summary has already been submitted for consideration of another Society (please specify).

7. A booklet of summaries will be available at the meeting. These summaries will be published unaltered in the British Journal of Surgery unless the Editorial Secretary is notified at the time of the meeting of any corrections which the author wishes to make to the summary.

    It is essential that the summary contains data with a clear description of the result and conlcusions; phrases such as "the results of these studies will be described" are not acceptable.

    The summary must closely follow the house style of the British Journal of Surgery. The British Journal of Surgery subscribes to the policy of Uniform Requirements for Manuscripts described in the British Medical Journal 1979; 1: 532-535 and Lancet 1979; 1: 428-431 which authors are advised to consult, and in the leaflet 'Uniform Requirements for Manuscripts Submitted to Biomedical Journals', which is available from the Editor, The British Medical Journal, BMA House, Tavistock Square, London, WC1.

    The title of the paper is typed in *lower case* and *single spacing* without the use of capitals except for the initial letter.

    Author(s) name(s) are typed in *capitals*.

    References should be kept to a minimum and must not exceed 4.

    In the text, references should be numbered consecutively in arabic numerals within parentheses (1 2 3...). The reference list is typed in numerical order.

All references cited should be listed according to the form of references adopted by Index Medicus. Up to six authors are listed; if the number exceeds six, quote the first three followed by et al. The sequence is author(s), title, journal, year, volume, first and last page numbers.

Books. Fuller details can be found in 'Uniform Requirements for Manuscripts submitted to Biomedical Journals' (International Steering Committee of Medical Editors) issued by the British Medical Journal.

8. **Textual Instructions**

   a) Items subsequently to be referred to in abbreviated form should be first indicated in full unless the abbreviation is an agreed one. Lists of agreed abbreviations will be circulated from time to time.

      - Abbreviations used to characterise animals (e.g. CBA, NZB) need not be explained in full.

      - Abbreviations are typed without full stops, e.g. DVT *not* D.V.T. (but lower case abbreviations have stops, e.g., s.e.m.).

      - Subscripts to abbreviations should not be used, e.g., PAO (Pg) is preferable to: PAO_{pg}

   b) Proper names should be used for drugs with, if more generally known, the trade name in brackets, e.g. aprotinin (Trasylol).

   c) S.I. nomenclature for quantities should be used wherever possible. Authors should refer to:

      - Quantities, Units and Symbols (1971), The Royal Society, London

      - Guide to Authors, Biochem. J. (1973), **131**, 1-20

      - Baron, D.N. (1974) S.I. Units, B.M.J., **4**, 509-512

9. Members who introduce papers are responsible for ensuring that summaries conform to these requirements.

10. Submission of summaries that do not conform to these requirements may result in the rejection of papers that are otherwise suitable.

SURGICAL RESEARCH SOCIETY

GUIDELINES FOR THE CONSTRUCTION AND USE OF SLIDES FOR SPEAKERS AT MEETINGS OF THE SURGICAL RESEARCH SOCIETY

GENERAL PRINCIPLES

1. Slides are illustrations and not aides memoires. Each one must give its message in four seconds; if attention is distracted from the speaker for any longer, it is not serving its purpose.

2. Tables make bad slides, and the same information can be better transmitted in the form of pie-charts, histograms, scattergrams or graphs.

3. Line drawings usually make better slides than photographs. Do not copy from books or papers, as there is always entraneous matter which must be eliminated before the material is suitable for presentation as a slide.

4. Do not read out what is on a slide (if the the audience is illiterate or the slide illegible, there is no point in showing it).

5. Usually no more than 8 slides are required for a 10-minute presentation.

DESIGN AND CONSTRUCTION

1. The size of a slide commonly accepted as standard is the 24×36mm format mounted in a 50×50 frame. Projection facilities for this size are universally available.

2. Information to be presented as a slide should be composed to fit a $2:3$ ratio.

3. Limit the number of words, data items and lines – a rough guide is the amount which can be typed onto a postcard 75×125mm using a 3mm typeface and double spacing.

4. Limit each slide to one main idea.

5. Select and simplify information. Use several slides rather than one which is complicated.

6. If the slide is to be referred to at different times in a lecture, have duplicates made.

7. Use a "blank" slide or a plain coloured slide rather than leave a slide on the screen when the topic is no longer being discussed.

8. Do not mix horizontal and vertical format slides when using either multiple projection or the "fade in" technique.

9. Do not pepper the text with capital letters – use either upper case or lower case consistently (except where proper names occur). Check all spelling and quotations, even when you feel sure you are right.

10. Avoid punctuation marks and underlining – create emphasis rather by the use of space and colour. If you do use lines make sure that they are the same width as the letters of the text. For drawings use China (matt) rather than India (gloss) ink and annotate horizontally, never vertically. Asterisks, squares or circles look more attractive than numbers before each sentence in a list.

11. Do not put letters, words or lines too close together. The optimum distances for text are: between letters, one-third of the height of the letter; between words, twice the width of a letter; and, between lines, one-and-a-half times the height of a letter.

12. Typing done on an electric typewriter using carbon ribbon and smooth surface paper will give good results particularly if a sans-serif typeface of 10-12 point and clean characters are used. Varafont 3000 or Letraset on A4 matt cartridge paper can be used with excellent results.

13. Lettering or artwork should be bold. Artwork on which typing is to be used should be about 90 × 120mm and not larger than 120 × 180mm.

USE OF SLIDES

1. Always hand film and slides to projectionist at the start of a meeting – not just when the paper is about to be presented.

2. Familiarise yourself with the lighting arrangements and the controls if projection is by remote control.

3. Mount slides carefully with a spot in the bottom left-hand corner.

4. Clean and check mounting of slides before each showing.

SURGICAL RESEARCH SOCIETY

ABBREVIATIONS LIST FOR S.R.S. SUMMARIES

Term General	Acceptable Abbreviation	Specification
Male	M	
Female	F	
Body weight	BW	kg

Statistical

Size of population	N	
Size of test subpopulation	n	
Probability	p	
Standard deviation	SD	
Standard error of mean	SEM	
Degrees of freedom	df	
Variance ratio	F	
Correlation coefficient	r	
"Student's" test	t test	
Standardised normal deviate	d	

Gastric Acid Tests

Basal acid output	BAO	Should be expressed in mmol/h
Maximal acid output	MAO	Acid output in the whole period 0-60 min. after a single parenteral injection of gastric stimulant, whether histamine, histalog, gastrin, tetragastrin or pentagastrin, should be expressed in mmol/h
Peak acid output	PAO	Acid output in the highest 2 consecutive 5, 10 or 15 min. collection periods after a single parenteral injection of gastric stimulant, whether histamine,

		histalog, gastrin, tetragastrin, pentagastrin or insulin, should be expressed in mmol/h
Plateau acid output	Plateau AO	Acid output in the highest 2 or more consecutive 5, 10 or 15 min. collection periods after an intravenous infusion of gastric stimulant, whether histamine, histalog, gastrin, tetragastrin, pentagastrin or insulin, should be expressed in mmol/h
Pentagastrin	Pg	
Maximum output after pentagastrin	MAO (pg)	
Peak acid output after pentagastrin	PAO (Pg)	
Peak acid output after insulin	PAO (I)	
Cholecystokinin	CCK	

Operations

Billroth I type partial gastrectomy	BI
Partial gastrectomy with gastrojejunal anastomosis	B II
Truncal vagotomy	TV
Selective vagotomy	SV
Highly selective vagotomy	HSV
Pyloroplasty (type not specified)	P
Pyloroplasty (Finney)	P (F)
Pyloroplasty (Heinecke-Mikulicz)	P (HM)
Gastroduodenostomy	GD
Gastrojejunostomy	GJ

INDEX